ANATOMY OF A COORDINATING COUNCIL

ERRATUM

Jacket and paper cover, second paragraph:
For Health Planning *Council* read Health Planning *Commission*

CONTEMPORARY COMMUNITY HEALTH SERIES

Titles in the Series

CHILDREN IN JEOPARDY

A Study of Abused Minors and Their Families

Elizabeth Elmer

EDUCATION AND MANPOWER
FOR COMMUNITY HEALTH

Hilary G. Fry, with the collaboration of
Ray H. Elling and William P. Shepard

HOME TREATMENT

Spearhead of Community Psychiatry

Leonard Weiner, Alvin Becker, and Tobias T. Friedman

MIGRANTS AND MALARIA IN AFRICA

R. Mansell Prothero

DENTISTS, PATIENTS, AND AUXILIARIES

Margaret Cussler and Evelyn W. Gordon

ANATOMY OF A COORDINATING COUNCIL

Implications for Planning

Basil J. F. Mott

ANATOMY OF A *Coordinating Council*

ANATOMY OF A *Coordinating Council*

Implications for Planning

---

by

BASIL J. F. MOTT

University of Pittsburgh Press

Library of Congress Catalog Card Number: 68–13934

Manufactured in the United States of America

This study is dedicated to the many New York State officials
who generously and frankly shared their views and
feelings about interdepartmental relations.
Their cooperation is a measure of their confidence
that progress in administrative affairs lies in impartial efforts
to fathom the realities of organizational life.

Contents

PART III

Evaluation and Conclusions

Tables

Foreword

PROFESSOR Mott's study deals with the coordinating process as it is embodied in the mechanism of an interagency committee at the state level in New York. Coordination is a venerable term, often used meaninglessly, seldom with precision. Broadly speaking, it means the reconciliation of conflicting objectives in common or interdependent activities. When the term refers to reorganization or bureaucratic reform, it is usually weighted with unexpressed values and objectives—with the supposition that centralization of power is good (or bad), with evaluations of programs that an organization should pursue (or ignore), or with the belief that duplication of effort is bad and, hence, that its elimination will provide a cheap and easy route to economy.

Coordination can include many political activities, but Professor Mott deals with interdepartmental coordination, which I take to mean increasing the compatibility of two or more bureaucratic units—a special case involving bureaucratic politics rather than the whole range of politics. This special case includes action by agency spokesmen whom we can expect to pursue relatively well-defined interests by recognizable means. It excludes political action by actors who do not know what they want or have little idea about how to get it. Characteristically, interdepartmental coordination proceeds without benefit of the strong authoritative relationships that one finds in the chain of command in centralized organizations. In Professor Mott's study, interdepartmental coordination occurs under the authority of the governor of New York, who has some legal powers to direct the agencies involved to follow common policies, but as a practical matter the governor remains mostly in the background. His participation and his effect on outcomes are much less than those of the U.S. President in regard to Cabinet business. Interdepartmental coordination in this study occurs in a relatively stable situation. The collectivities whose interests are represented in the committee are not temporary political factions or groups that spring into existence over some issue and later dissolve. They are formal, more or less stable organizations with a past and a future.

Coordination also occurs within formal organizations and among relatively autonomous organizations not subordinate to a common authority. The degree of interdependence among the coordinated units and the strength of the central authority over them—if any—are the two most important variables affecting the achievement of coordination. In Professor Mott's study of the Interdepartmental Health and Hospital Council, these two variables are represented respectively by the departments of a larger organization (the executive branch of the state, headed by the governor) and the legal powers that the governor himself exercises over these departments.

The literature on interdepartmental coordination in public administration is neither theoretically rich nor empirically precise. Its weakness invites improvement. A promising way to improve it would be to order and explain data from a wider range of findings about political and behavioral phenomena. Professor Mott's study is a valuable addition to such findings.

Studies of interagency coordination in U.S. public administration have focused mainly on overall coordination of federal activities. Before the New Deal the major writings on interdepartmental coordination were concerned with the executive budget movement, which became linked with the drive for strong executive authority in local, state, and national government. At the federal level this movement was part of the effort to achieve economy and efficiency, which gained impetus under the Taft Administration, but it did not achieve much of practical consequence until the enactment of the Budget and Accounting Act of 1921. Interdepartmental coordination then became strongly identified with the process of executive budgeting. In 1939, the staff agency which presided over this process on behalf of the President—the Bureau of the Budget—became a sort of superagency with broad responsibilities for coordinating departmental activities for the President.

Much of the early writing about this executive budget process was explanatory and hortatory. For example, President Taft, in explaining the purpose of his Commission on Economy and Efficiency, set as an objective better government as well as cheaper government, yet such efforts were broader in purpose and objective than the economy-minded reorganization efforts in the post-World War II period.[1]

A study of interdepartmental committees by Mary T. Reynolds,[2] published in 1939, when the Bureau of the Budget was assuming greater responsibilities on behalf of the President, concentrated on better government. The work is topical and pedestrian. Occasionally it develops and applies some functional categories that might be worth exploring further, but does not make any cumulative application of them. However, it does consider the question: How much coordination is a good thing? "Complete reconciliation of all interests will be impossible; agreements can only be temporary and imperfect," Miss Reynolds argued. "Moreover, as government moves through different phases of a program, a later decision may cancel out an earlier. Contingency must be counted as an important factor in both legislative and administrative planning."[3] This pragmatic and incremental view of the governmental process treated coordination as a nondefinable value.

The upgrading of the Bureau of the Budget and other steps

1. President Taft is quoted in Jesse Burkhead, *Government Budgeting* (New Work: Wiley, 1956), p. 19. See also *Message of the President of the United States on Economy and Efficiency in the Government Service, with Appendix*, H. Doc. 458, 62nd Cong., 2d Sess. (1912). The postwar trend from better government to cheaper government is described and condemned in Edward A. Fitzpatrick, *Budget Making in a Democracy: A New View of the Budget* (New York: Macmillan, 1918), pp. 1–23.

2. *Interdepartmental Committees in the National Administration* (New York: Columbia U. Press, 1939).

3. *Ibid.*, p. 163.

taken to strengthen the President's staff are reflected in the 1937 report of the findings of the Brownell Committee.[4] The Committee was a group of experts on management and government from outside the government, who shared the vision of a strong political executive that had inspired the municipal reform movement at the turn of the century. Centralized executive power, which had looked attractive to young Republicans during Theodore Roosevelt's Administration, and which had seemed to follow the lead of the great business corporations established in the late nineteenth century, became a model for New Deal Democrats in the thirties, who found the Chief Executive more receptive to their views and demands than Congress or the state governments.

Mobilization in two world wars produced valuable experience in interdepartmental coordination in Washington. Most serious publications on the subject coming out of World War I[5] were heavily prescriptive, but they provided some accurate descriptions of coordination and control techniques, usually without adequately accounting for political factors.

Partisan Republicans prodded President Wilson with reorganization proposals during World War I. The attitudes that had legitimized energetic government as well as big business under Theodore Roosevelt and Taft became, in World War I, a weapon used by the Republicans against Wilson. The war effort on the home front, they contended, should be directed by a businessman "czar," who would take mobilization out of politics. Administrative literature, however, has neglected the broad impact and very considerable political dimensions of the somewhat jerry-built

4. President's Committee on Administrative Management, *Report with Special Studies* (Washington: Government Printing Office, 1937.

5. Daniel R. Beaver, *Newton D. Baker and the American War Effort, 1917–1919* (Lincoln: U. of Nebraska Press, 1966); Bernard M. Baruch, *American Industry in the War: A Report of the War Industries Board* (New York: Prentice-Hall, 1941); Major General Johnson Hagood, *The Services of Supply* (Boston: Houghton Mifflin, 1923); Benedict Crowell and Robert F. Wilson, *The Giant Hand: Our Mobilization and Control of Industry and Natural Resources, 1917–1918* (New Haven: Yale U. Press, 1921).

superagencies and interdepartmental coordinating devices used in the Wilson Administration.

By contrast, the World War II coordinating experiences, which came on top of the New Deal coordinating efforts, have been amply described.[6] They have also been illuminatingly analyzed in a major source, Herman Somers' book on the principal (though by no means exclusive) coordinating agency for the home front, the Office of War Mobilization and Reconversion.[7]

After World War II, writings on federal coordinating experiences were based on the assumption that coordination within the executive branch was a much needed thing, and that it would improve executive-congressional relations.[8] The National Security Council, an outgrowth of Franklin Roosevelt's disorderly executive style in World War II, reflected this outlook in its origins, though not entirely in its development. President Truman, correctly detecting that its sponsors intended to "organize" the President out of some of his discretion, was cool toward the Council until the Korean War.[9]

President Eisenhower used the National Security Council to produce a more orderly process of coordination in the White

6. For a full bibliographical treatment see Committee on Civil-Military Relations Research, Social Science Research Council, *Civil-Military Relations: An Annotated Bibliography, 1940–1952* (New York: Columbia U. Press, 1954), Chap. 8.

7. Herman M. Somers, *Presidential Agency: OWMR, the Office of War Mobilization and Reconversion* (Cambridge: Harvard U. Press, 1950).

8. Daniel S. Cheever and H. Field Haviland, Jr., *American Foreign Policy and the Separation of Powers* (Cambridge: Harvard U. Press, 1952); and the [first Hoover] Commission on Organization of the Executive Branch of the Government, *Task Force Report on National Security Organization,* (Washington: Government Printing Office, 1949), and *Task Force Report on the Federal Supply System* (1949), esp. pp. 25–26.

9. A fairly recent summary of the Council's activities will be found in Stanley L. Falk, "The National Security Council Under Truman, Eisenhower, and Kennedy," *Political Science Qtly.*, LXXIX (Sept. 1964), 403–34. See also Senate Government Operations Committee, *Conduct of National Security Policy, Part 1*, Hearings, 89th Cong., 1st Sess. (1965), p. 43; "Organizational History of the National Security Council," in SGOC, *Organizing for National Security*, 87th Cong., 1st Sess. (1966), pp. 411–68.

House. There is some dispute as to the results. The most candid, if not the most balanced, memoir of the Eisenhower years flatly claims that chaos prevailed.[10] Other evidence confirms the view that the procedures of the Eisenhower White House, both in domestic and foreign affairs, were often overloaded with trivia and failed to deal with the main issues of the Presidency. Attempts to explain this situation emphasize the fact that Cabinet members were usually able to deal with the President only individually, rather than at Cabinet meetings or through the National Security Council.[11] There is a similarity here to the permissive attitude of the governor in Professor Mott's study in allowing his department heads to have access to him personally. The Cabinet officers and other members of the Eisenhower Administration, however, were able to approach the President only through the channels afforded by his staff system. As a result, his Cabinet officers developed a propensity, when acting on business at the Cabinet level, to neglect the President's interests and perspectives.[12]

During the Kennedy and Johnson Administrations, federal interdepartmental coordination has reflected the increased interest in programs of greater breadth and variety for dealing with domestic problems and in programs for developing a more cohesive (coordinated) administration of foreign affairs. The coordination of domestic programs has taken two forms. First, new programs have been drawn across department lines, generating new problems of coordination among agencies. In the War on Poverty—the out-

10. Emmet John Hughes, *The Ordeal of Power: A Political Memoir of the Eisenhower Years* (New York: Atheneum, 1963), Chaps. 3 and 4.

11. Richard F. Fenno, Jr., *The President's Cabinet* (Cambridge: Harvard U. Press, 1959), *passim.*

12. Arthur M. Schlesinger, Jr., *The Coming of the New Deal* (Boston: Houghton Mifflin, 1959), pp. 518–20, and 522 ff; Richard E. Neustadt, *Presidential Power: The Politics of Leadership* (New York: Wiley, 1960), esp. Chap. 6; Paul Y. Hammond, "The National Security Council as a Device for Interdepartmental Coordination: An Interpretation and Appraisal," *American Political Science Rev.*, LIV (Dec. 1960), 899–910; Arthur Maass, "Protecting Nature's Reservoir," in *Public Policy,* ed. C. J. Friedrich and J. K. Galbraith (Cambridge: Harvard Graduate School of Public Administration, 1954), V (1954), 71–106.

standing example—the Office of Economic Opportunity, located in the Executive Office of the President, is charged with supervising and coordinating activities in several major executive departments.[13] As with much of the New Deal administrative superstructure, the administrative experience in the War on Poverty has been dominated by rapidly changing political factors. It is a "system-dominant subsystem," so to speak, and inferences about it are difficult to draw because the major determinants of behavior lie outside the subsystem.

The second method of coordinating domestic federal programs consists of regrouping activities in new major executive departments on the basis of outputs (programs and functions) rather than inputs (the servicing of compatible interest groups or clienteles). The Department of Health, Education, and Welfare was the first of these new departments. It was followed by the Department of Housing and Urban Development and the Department of Transportation. There was also the surprising attempt of the Johnson Administration to combine the Commerce and Labor Departments—surprising because, on the input side, the labor and business clientele groups are staunch adversaries and thus were fiercely opposed to the proposal—but consistent with the output concept behind the three new departments. Agencies set up to supervise, regulate, promote, or protect a private clientele develop strong interdependent relationships with such clienteles. Often the agencies are captured by their clients (a common criticism, for example, of the Federal Communications Commission and the Interstate Commerce Commission), or they acquire considerable autonomy (well-known examples are the Army Corps of Engineers, the Federal Bureau of Investigation, and the Children's Bureau, which, though its former autonomy has been well de-

13. The administrative arrangements of the Office of Economic Opportunity are briefly described in Senate Labor and Public Welfare Committee, *Examination of the War on Poverty,* Hearings, 90th Cong., 1st. Sess. (1967), Part 10, pp. 3388–3406. The coordination problem is discussed in Office of Economic Opportunity, *The Quiet Revolution* (Washington: Government Printing Office, 1967), pp. 79–85.

scribed,[14] is no longer as independent as it once was). Any public agency confronts potential clientele groups with at least some objectives that exceed the particular interests of the groups. The new generation of executive departments is noted for the degree to which their functions cut across and transcend the interests of their clientele groups. This gives the departments an advantage in that it helps them to avoid captivity and "privatization" of their policies. Indeed, a minimum requirement for a public agency (as distinct from a private one) in the performance of its functions is that it not have a one-to-one relationship with any of its clientele groups. "Before-and-after" studies of the performance of the functions of these new departments, comparing the ways in which the same functions were previously performed, would be highly informative in regard to the coordination process, but as yet no such studies have been produced.

The Kennedy and Johnson Administrations also attempted to improve interdepartmental administration of foreign relations.[15] President Kennedy's main contribution was the emphasis given to the ambassador as head of a team that included not only State Department personnel in the embassy of the country involved and in State Department-administered agencies, such as the Agency for International Development and the U.S. Information Agency, but also personnel representing other departments, such as members of the Military Assistance Advisory Groups and even officials of the Veterans Administration. The Johnson Administration brought this "country-team" concept to Washington and established a structure of interdepartmental committees, including country subcommittees (usually headed by the Country Director from the State Department), interregional groups (headed by regional Assistant Secretaries of State), and a government-wide committee at the deputy or undersecretary level (headed by the

14. See "The Transfer of the Children's Bureau," in *Public Administration and Policy Development*, ed. Harold Stein (New York: Harcourt, Brace, 1952), pp. 15–30.

15. Senate Government Operations Committee, *The Secretary of State and the Problem of Coordination*, Committee Print, 89th Cong., 2d Sess. (1966).

Undersecretary of State). However, as late as 1967, only the inter-regional group for Latin America had shown any evidence of life. Some studies of these efforts have been circulating within the government, and doubtless published reports will soon be forthcoming.

So far we have considered interagency coordination of the type in which the methods and the incentives have involved accommodation of interests without special reference to the criteria for accommodation, largely because objective criteria have not been important elements in the accommodation process. But important strides have been made and reported in interagency coordination in which the coordination process has involved analytical criteria and methods.

The *executive budget* was the first recognized example of interagency coordination by the analytical method. Later developments of the executive budget were *program budgeting,* which had a vogue in the late forties and early fifties, and the *systems concept,* developed as a management tool in the fifties.[16] A recent, much-heralded attempt at coordination by the analytical method is the effort to develop a government-wide *programming, planning, and budgeting system.* This system, known by its acronym, PPBS, was modeled after the Department of Defense management revolution of the early 1960's. It is an impressive effort to generate analytical methods for interdepartmental coordination[17] and a highly refined application of program budgeting methods that

16. Arthur Smithies reflects the contemporary popularity of program budgeting in his *The Budgetary Process in the United States* (New York: McGraw-Hill, 1955), esp. Chap. 11. Frederick C. Mosher questions it in his *Program Budgeting: Theory and Practice* (Chicago: Public Administration Service, 1954), and more recently in "PPBS: Two Questions," reprinted in Senate Government Operations Committee, *Planning Programming-Budgeting,* Committee Print, 90th Cong., 1st Sess. (1967), pp. 23–28.

17. Gene H. Fisher makes this point in "The Role of Cost-Utility Analysis in Program Budgeting," Chap. 3 of *Program Budgeting,* ed. David Novick (Cambridge: Harvard U. Press, 1965), p. 63. This volume and C. J. Hitch and R. N. McKean, eds., *The Economics of Defense in the Nuclear Age* (Cambridge: Harvard U. Press, 1960), are standard though introductory works on the analytical methods, processes, and components of PPBS.

have been in use in the Department of Defense and elsewhere in the federal government for many years.[18] The Defense Comptroller's staff superimposed upon a statute-based system of accounts (broken down by armed services—Army, Navy, Air Force) estimated cost accounts aggregated according to nine basic department programs. They then locked these programs into both a short-run budget allocation system and a five-year planning effort, and added to the system (but not to the actual budget) the costs of nuclear warheads and bombs, even though nuclear weapons are funded through the Atomic Energy Commission.

The executive budget, the program budget, and PPBS all make it possible, by the way they keep accounts and organize data, for management to view the relationship of the agency's input to its output in terms other than formal structure and sometimes in several different terms. They provide management with different views of the organization, usually by arranging data on operations into representations of the organization's inputs, processes, and outputs, as the outputs relate to specific programs. It is principally a matter of sorting and manipulating information: Cost analysis is a way of generating the information to be sorted; systems analysis, a way of generating and manipulating information in order to present graphically the subjects or programs that management wishes to examine. This combination of cost analysis and systems analysis, by increasing the data base and providing a means for converting data into pictures of operations, has made it possible for management to multiply the number of views it can have and the ways in which it can act upon what it manages.

One drawback of the program budgeting proposals of the mid-

18. David Novick traces it back to the 1942 Controlled Materials Plan of the War Production Board in his "Origin and History of Program Budgeting" (RAND Corp. Paper No. P–3427, Oct. 1966), pp. 1–5. But the Controlled Materials Plan has some kinship to the material control system administered by Bernard Baruch in World War I. (See his *American Industry in the War*, Note 5, above). Novick refers to program budgeting in DuPont and General Motors at least as early as 1924. Possibly the wartime experience in 1919 in Washington can be related to this corporation experience in Wilmington and Detroit in the early twenties.

fifties was that they paid little attention to the reasons why the programs advocated were better than existing or alternative programs.[19] More recently, a similar problem has arisen in systems analysis—the failure, when designing a system model, to take into account the predictable outcome that the design will be modified or superseded within a few years.[20] The PPBS approach is also beset with obstacles, many undoubtedly insurmountable. For example, a PPBS system for the State Department or for foreign affairs generally, should in principle take account of activities important to foreign affairs regardless of what agency funds these activities, as has been done in the defense sector. However, no such system as yet exists, and efforts to develop one in 1965 were disappointing. They were described in a case study by Frederick C. Mosher and John O. Harr.[21]

Moreover, PPBS is not simply an analytic methodology. Though often presented by its advocates and practitioners as an unbiased (or value neutral) aid to decision-making, it clearly gives weight to tangible and quantifiable values (especially those of welfare economics) at the expense of others and, in the tradition of the economy and efficiency movement from which it partly springs, has a marked aversion to politics. Yet its application implies centralization of power and authority and thus fundamental changes in the operation of the political process.[22] But the successful use of PPBS in the Department of Defense and the persistence of interdepartmental coordination problems of both foreign and domestic affairs strongly suggest that great efforts will be made to

19. F. C. Mosher, *Program Budgeting: Theory and Practice,* pp. 236 ff. Mosher has recently lamented the lack of historical perspective about program budgeting in his "PPBS: Two Questions," p. 27.

20. See especially James R. Schlesinger, "The Changing Environment for Systems Analysis" (RAND Corp., Paper No. P–3287, Dec. 1965), also Schlesinger, "Organization Structures and Planning" (RAND Corp., Paper No. P–3316, Feb. 25, 1966), and "On Relating Non-Technical Elements to System Studies" (RAND Corp., Paper No. P–3545, Feb. 1967).

21. Inter-University Case Program, "Program Budgeting Visits Foreign Affairs: A Case Study," Syracuse, 1967 (mimeo.).

22. Aaron Wildavsky, "The Political Economy of Efficiency," *The Public Interest* (Summer, 1967), pp. 30–48.

develop PPBS and to compensate for its limitations.

The implementation of the coordination process by analytical methods takes other forms than those related to the budgetary process. In any form, the analysis usually depends on some quantitative methods. Probably the most successful analytical coordinative function (one with highly developed quantitative components) has been performed by the Council of Economic Advisors. Since its establishment in 1946 it has become the producer of high-quality, modern, economic macroanalyses of the major policy issues faced by the President in managing the national economy. Unmistakably, the Council operates in a political environment, but the remarkable growth of its influence is largely due to the technical capabilities it has acquired by exploiting the increasing number of analytical tools of modern economics.[23]

Analytical methods of coordination take their strength from their capacity to deal with the substance of issues rather than simply to provide an arena in which interests can be accommodated. The more rigorous the analysis, the wider the area of agreement has to be in the first place. The coordination of Defense Department policies by methods of analysis was possible because of the existence in 1961 of a foundation of techniques and concepts developed over the previous decade or so, largely in the semiprivate sector of defense contractors, and largely unexploited to that date. Coordination was also aided by the existence of an impressive accounting system, which provided an infrastructure of data, so to speak, and by the existence of strong though hitherto unasserted statutory powers residing in the Secretary of Defense, who used them to take the initiative and thereby kept opposition from forming around rival analytical methods.[24]

So far we have considered interagency coordination at the federal level only. From this level we can go "up," "down," or "out."

23. Edward S. Flash, Jr., *Economic Advice and Presidential Leadership* (New York: Columbia U. Press, 1965), esp. pp. 269–74.

24. Paul Y. Hammond, "A Functional Analysis of Defense Department Decision-Making," *American Political Science Rev.*, LXI (March 1968).

By "up" I mean to the international level. What is regarded in any one country as U.S. foreign policy can be taken as the accommodation of two or more rather complex organizations—our foreign office and theirs, our embassy and their government, our mission and several other missions. In this area of coordination the writing is diverse. There are studies of techniques used in formal negotiations; there are commentaries and memoirs about diplomacy[25] and elaborate and illuminating studies about the accommodation process and its environment.[26] Here, the relationship of agencies to each other is sometimes altered by design to make the whole process of accommodation easier. It is a special case of political integration in which the principal driving force is usually success at interdepartmental coordination, either by technical analysis or accommodative bargaining.

By "out" I mean to the level at which interdepartmental committees in other governments operate, such as the British Committee of Imperial Defense.[27] Here the opportunities for making comparative studies of interagency coordination are plainly immense.

By "down" I mean to state and local levels and finally to a level represented by another corpus of serious writing—on competition, cooperation, and collusion, which are forms of coordination among business firms. States often have been run at the highest level by committees that are somewhat like a mayor-council form of government: an elected governor, sitting with from three to six

25. Fred C. Iklé in *How Nations Negotiate* (New York: Harper and Row, 1964) codifies and analyzes hostile negotiations; C. Turner Joy's *How Communists Negotiate* (New York: Macmillan, 1955) is an example of a memoir that analyzes techniques; Robert Murphy's *Diplomat among Warriers* (Garden City: Doubleday, 1964) exemplifies the memoir in more traditional form, in which diplomatic techniques are a subject of comment *en passant*.

26. Ernest B. Haas, *Beyond the Nation-State* (Stanford: Stanford U. Press, 1964), pp. 3–125. For a description of the integration process and, tangentially, its effect on policy coordination, see Haas, *The Uniting of Europe* (Stanford: Stanford U. Press, 1958), esp. pp. 241–280.

27. Franklyn A. Johnson, *Defense by Committee* (London: Oxford U. Press, 1960).

other elected officials, each controlling some segment of state government. Most of the literature on these state committees or governor's councils is too preoccupied with telling us that they work badly to concern itself with how they work at all. Professor Mott's study concerns a governor's council, but it is one step "down" from a governor's cabinet. It is the only major published study, so far as I know, to concern itself with this level of state government—and it is not at all preoccupied with telling us how bad the real world of state government is.

Further "down," at the local government level are works that range from reports on the sprawling pluralism of megalopolis, as represented by New York City and Chicago, to reports on the personal interactions of town finance committees in Connecticut.[28] The coordination of political efforts in Chicago is dealt with by Banfield, who calls the complex structures of influence that he describes "concerting action by influence."[29] He allows for the high number of relatively independent political actors and treats their efforts at coordination in terms of the techniques and incentives of politicians. Sayre and Kaufman's massive study of New York City[30] deals with the techniques of political influence that are exploitable by individual actors or groups (including agencies) and with the broadest patterns of competitive and aggregative relationships. Dahl[31] concerns himself with the integration of the actions of various political leaders.

Once we have included in our ambit not only the behavior of

28. James David Barber, *Power In Committees* (Chicago: Rand McNally, 1966). This book reports a laboratory study of real government bodies—town finance committees in Connecticut. For a report on the experimental study of coordinating groups see A. Zander and D. Wolfe, "Administrative Rewards and Coordination Among Committee Members," *Administrative Science Qtly.*, IX (June 1964), pp. 50–69.

29. This is the title of chapter twelve of Edward C. Banfield, *Political Influence* (New York: Free Press, 1962), p. 307.

30. Wallace S. Sayre and H. Kaufman, *Governing New York City: Politics in the Metropolis* (New York: Russell Sage Foundation, 1960), *passim* and Chap. 19.

31. Robert A. Dahl, *Who Governs?* (New Haven: Yale U. Press, 1962).

federal and state interdepartmental groups but program budgeting, diplomacy, metropolitan political life, and the personal interactions of town finance committees, not much is left. What has been said so far, however, should make clear that interdepartmental committees—and any of these other groups or situations—are all special cases of coordination.

If we take coordination to be the integration or harmonization of efforts, then the analytical issues can be stated schematically in the following way: Coordination is accomplished by influence, which takes different forms in different situations. The two principal forms are authoritative direction and mutual accommodation. Analytical methods of coordination can be adapted to either the directive or the accommodative form.[32] Situations can be classified according to the degree of integration among units. The integration can be both social and structural; structural integration can be either lateral or hierarchical (giving rise to accommodative and directive forms of coordination, respectively). Autonomy, the opposite of integration, can vary in expression from competitive relationships found within a common bureaucracy to hostile relationships among nation-states, such as those

32. Analytical methods that have proved useful in coordinative mechanisms depend on economic theory—in the same way that game theory depends on studies of market competition and other economic models. Thomas C. Schelling's *The Strategy of Conflict* (Cambridge: Harvard U. Press, 1960) presents an approach to coordinated political behavior that uses broad analogues. Kenneth Arrow and L. Hurwitz, in "Decentralization and Computation in Resource Allocation" (*Studies in Mathematical Economics and Econometrics,* ed. R. W. Phoutts, Chapel Hill: U. of N. Carolina Press, 1962), Thomas Marschak, in "Economic Theories of Organization" (*Handbook of Organizations,* ed. James E. March, Chicago: Rand McNally, 1965), and Martin Shubik, in *Oligopoly, Competition, and the Theory of Games* (New York: Wiley, 1959) represent a more precise and less concrete handling of this varied domain. Community political studies, at least those written by political scientists, reflect the market orientation of economic studies—and the debt such studies owe to classical economics. The most comprehensive adaptation of marketplace literature to coordination is to be found in Charles E. Lindblom, *The Intelligence of Democracy* (New York: Free Press, 1965).

between military establishments. (In the latter case, coordination would be represented by arms control.)

There is no single all-embracing mechanism for the accomplishment of coordination. For example, the organizational and political processes (authoritative direction, mutual accommodation) by which coordination is accomplished within a small, unified, well-led agency with strong clientele support are different from the processes by which it is achieved among agencies that lack effective clientele support and (possibly) effective leadership. Drawing generalizations is therefore a risky business, but a still more formidable obstacle to our understanding of the coordinating process up to now has been the mediocre quality of the investigations reported and a need for research in all types of coordination.

Professor Mott has helped to correct this deficiency by thoroughly investigating a particular mechanism, created for the primary purpose of effecting coordination. By exploring fully the broader implications of his study, he also has delineated many issues central to an understanding of the processes of coordination and to an understanding of organizational and political life in general.

PAUL Y. HAMMOND
Rand Corporation

Preface

ALL who work in organizations, whether they are heads of agencies, middle managers, or technical and clerical personnel, perform their tasks constrained by impersonal forces of which they often are unaware. These fundamental organizational factors, which limit one's freedom of action and even shape one's perceptions, have long been poorly understood, if recognized at all. Only in recent years have students of organization—scholars and reflective administrators—begun to grasp them.

Coordination of the programs of different health agencies is an important area in which lack of knowledge of the operation of these underlying factors has been especially marked. Health adminstrators and the elected officials to whom they are accountable often have sought through various cooperative arrangements to bring about coordination among agencies, little recognizing the forces inherent in such situations that prevent agency heads and their staffs from fulfilling the goals sought. They have not, for example, appreciated that the behavior of agency officials is constrained by the need for their agencies to pursue policies that will assure them sufficient resources to maintain themselves as viable organizations (funds, manpower, facilities, and other support).

Thus, it has generally been overlooked that an agency head and his staff are unable to engage in cooperative endeavors with other organizations that threaten the agency's future and its capacity to meet the public needs to which its members and supporters are committed. Every public agency necessarily adopts a view of the public interest that reconciles its organizational needs with the needs of those it serves; this conception governs its relations with other organizations. However, even when there has been awareness of these necessities, there has been a tendency to regard them uncritically as responses to "vested interests." Consequently, when interagency coordinating and planning bodies have been established, there has been too little understanding of how they must operate and what can reasonably be expected of them. Similarly, there has been an inclination to judge their performance by inappropriate criteria, and thus either to overrate or underrate their effectiveness.

In this study of a succession of New York State interdepartmental health councils, Professor Mott makes an important contribution to knowledge of interagency relationships in general and to understanding of interagency coordinating and planning councils in particular. By probing deeply for the underlying variables that explain why the councils operated as they did, he does much to clarify the organizational factors governing relations among agencies having interrelated programs. Much of the value of the study comes from fruitful application of modern concepts of organization. The analysis is also executed with appreciation of the nuances of behavior in bureaucratic agencies. As a health administrator and teacher, I find that the most important contributions of the study are its demonstration that a coordinating mechanism without authority can achieve only a very limited degree of coordination and that the problem of achieving coordination among different health agencies having related functions is fundamentally a question of designing organizational arrangements that are suitable to the task at hand. I am convinced that "coordinates" cannot coordinate each other when they must compete for the same things. Although the leadership and administrative skills of health leaders are important in attaining coordination, they cannot make an inadequate organizational structure work effectively.

This is not to dismiss the importance of leadership and the personal skills of gifted administrators. These attributes are important, but health administrators have overemphasized these factors at the expense of others. If community health experts are to continue to meet effectively the changing health needs of a growing population, they must see clearly that there are intrinsic elements in all organizational situations that determine what any administrator can accomplish. Progress in organizational affairs lies in recognizing these factors and learning how to deal with them. The era of comprehensive community health that we now are entering makes it all the more important for us to become masters of organization and management, which means better understanding the limits of our control as administrators.

Professor Mott's study of interdepartmental councils has given me a new insight of considerable depth and clarity and an objective view that I did not have when I was personally involved with these councils over a span of sixteen years. We are certain to have more interdepartmental health councils in the future; this study should help us avoid some of the old pitfalls.

HERMAN E. HILLEBOE, M.D.
De Lamar Professor
of Public Health Practice

Acknowledgments

AUTHORSHIP usually rests on the cooperation of others. This study is no exception.

I especially wish to express my appreciation to Herman E. Hilleboe, M.D., of Columbia University, and James Q. Wilson of Harvard University for their critical review of the manuscript in each of its several drafts and for their personal encouragement from the inception of the project.

I also want to acknowledge my indebtedness to a friend and former colleague, William Thomas, Jr., of Columbia University, for his perceptive advice, to Sol Levine of Johns Hopkins University, for his valuable suggestions, and to the New York State officials whom I interviewed and who generously provided access to records and meetings—in particular Edward R. Schlesinger, M.D., formerly of the State Department of Health, and Paul E. Robinson and Joseph Fenton, formerly of the Staff of the Interdepartmental Health and Hospital Council.

Finally, I owe a large debt to a special friend, Michael Lesparre of the American Hospital Association, for expert editing of the manuscript, and to Mrs. Anita Gourley for her exceptional loyalty and patience as a secretary.

The research on which this manuscript is based was financed by funds provided to the School of Public Health and Administrative Medicine of Columbia University by the New York State Department of Health on behalf of the New York State Interdepartmental Health and Hospital Council.

ANATOMY OF A
Coordinating Council

Introduction

INTERAGENCY coordinating councils are a familiar feature of the American scene, yet not much has been learned about them in a systematic way. Although they are one of the most common mechanisms by which interagency planning (joint determination of ends and means) and less threatening forms of interorganizational accommodation are pursued, there has been surprisingly little reporting and less analysis of the operation of such councils.[1] Most studies have dealt with individual organizations rather than the relations among organizations.[2] Consequently, present knowl-

1. See Chap. 1 and the Bibliography.

2. Amitai Etzioni points out that "only in the last few years have organizational studies turned to systematic examination of the relations between organizations and external social units [including interrelations among organizations]." See "New Directions in the Study of Organizations and Society," *Social Research,* XXVII (Summer 1960), 223. Sol Levine and Paul E. White report that "studies of interrelationships have largely been confined to units within the same organizational structure or between a pair of complementary organizations such as management and labor." See "Exchange as a Conceptual Framework for the Study of Interorganizational Relationships," *Administrative Science Qtly.,* V (March 1961), 584. Eugene Litwak and Lydia F. Hylton suggest that "one major lacuna in current sociological study is research on interorganizational relations—studies which use organizations as their unit of analysis." See "Interorganizational Analysis: A Hypothesis on Coordinating Agencies," *Administrative Science Qtly.,* VI (March 1962), 395.

edge offers little to guide the man of affairs or the student of organization interested in the underlying theoretical questions.

This study is intended to learn something about the operation of interagency councils or committees: How do they handle conflicts of interest among their members? Under what conditions do the member agencies engage in cooperative behavior? How is their operation affected by the organizational needs of the member agencies? How are such mechanisms influenced by environmental factors? In what ways are they effective or ineffective instrumentalities? The purpose of the inquiry, which employs the case study method, is twofold: (1) to describe, analyze, and appraise the operation of a particular council, and (2) in so doing, to illuminate some of the organizational exigencies that influence the functioning of coordinating councils. A major objective is the development of a fruitful approach for the analysis of such instrumentalities and to suggest hypotheses that may explain their performance. This aspect of the study is exploratory.

There are many different formal mechanisms by which the activities of separate organizations are coordinated (concerted for some purpose). Coordinating councils, which typically have little or no formal authority over their members, are distinguished from hierarchical coordinating structures, such as governors' offices, executive budget offices, and central planning bodies, in which superior-subordinate relationships, and thus formal authority, are a central means of control. Although there is a wide variety of coordinating councils (including, for example, the community planning councils common in the health and welfare field and the many interdepartmental committees found at all levels of government), characteristically they are peer groups having little or no formal authority to compel their members to accept their decisions. Thus they constitute a distinct organizational form that warrants special study. The increasing importance of formal organizations in our society also makes the subject of interorganizational coordination of vital and growing significance. As organized group effort becomes more important and specialized, our lives inevitably become more interdependent.

The subject of this study is the Interdepartmental Health and Hospital Council (IHHC) of New York State.[3] This council was selected primarily because it offered a strong example—unlike many coordinating councils, it showed many signs of success. The Council was active for two decades and spanned three state administrations; it had a high degree of acceptance by the participants and others concerned with it. For example, the representatives of the member agencies and governors and their aides generally considered it one of the most effective bodies of its kind in the state government. The Council's operation also was marked by an extraordinary high degree of attendance by the heads of member agencies. Finally, as a practical matter, the Council was accessible to the author because of the interest of state officials in learning more about its performance.

The study deals with the operation of the Council as a whole; however in several chapters, particularly those dealing with the subordinate levels at which the Council linked the member agencies and the effectiveness of the instrumentality, it focuses more upon coordination of state rehabilitation programs for the handicapped than upon the Council's operation in other program sectors. Moreover, such quantitative data as it has been possible to use have been drawn from the area of rehabilitation.

Methodological and practical considerations fortuitously converged. According to almost everyone familiar with the Council,

3. The Interdepartmental Health and Hospital Council (IHHC) was the third and last name of a coordinating council originally created by Governor Thomas E. Dewey on October 5, 1946, as the Interdepartmental Health Council (IHC), which continued under that name until March 31, 1956, when Governor W. Averell Harriman broadened its scope and renamed it the Interdepartmental Health Resources Board (IHRB). The IHRB continued in existence until March 31, 1960, when Governor Nelson A. Rockefeller supplanted it with the Interdepartmental Health and Hospital Council (IHHC), which went out of existence on June 30, 1967, its functions being assumed by the New York State Health Planning Commission. Throughout this study the coordinating council, regardless of its phase or name at any given time, will be referred to as *the Council*, unless it is necessary to pinpoint a specific phase, in which case the appropriate name or acronym—*IHC*, *IHRB*, or *IHHC*—will be used.

it was most active and successful in the area of rehabilitation. Consequently, examination of the Council's functioning in this program sector shows the mechanism at its best. Objective indications also support this judgment. For example, the Committee on Rehabilitation met more frequently (monthly) over a longer period of time (12 years) than any other Council committee; on the whole its meetings were among the best attended; and finally, the Council had more to show for its efforts in this area than in any other.[4] Also, rehabilitation is truly an interdepartmental activity. Although it might be possible to combine some of the rehabilitation programs of the member agencies, they could not all be united in a single agency. Furthermore, in order to study Council operations at three levels (Council proper, central committee, and regional committee), it is necessary to concentrate on rehabilitation, as it is the only program sector in which the mechanism spawned regional interdepartmental committees.[5] Moreover, the state sponsors of the research were particularly interested in examining and assessing the Council's performance in coordinating New York's rehabilitation programs.

As a case study, the research is concerned with discerning the operating characteristics of an organization of organizations that attempts to coordinate relations among its members without benefit of formal authority. The concern therefore is with the behavior of individuals as organizational representatives or, in other words, with those aspects of their behavior that are determined by organizational considerations in contradistinction to differences in personality.[6] It is of course recognized that indi-

4. Covers the period 1953–1964. More current data show that this pattern continued through the life of the Council. See pp. 39–42.

5. The Committee on Coordination of School and Community Health Services, 1946–1953, also developed regional committees, but they were ill-defined and came to naught, mainly because of underlying disagreement among the member agencies over their functions. By contrast, the regional rehabilitation committees represented a continuing and much more highly developed effort to foster coordination.

6. As Victor A. Thompson says: "Organization theory is not concerned with personality. Personality theory attempts to account for variations in

vidual motives and idiosyncracies have an effect on organizational destinies. However, some loss in completeness is accepted in order to gain the larger benefit of elucidating the organizational regularities. Similarly, the study is not concerned with substantive questions of policy and administration, except as the Council's impact upon state policies and programs tells us something about its behavior and characteristics as an organizational structure.

The study is divided into three parts: (1) a section on basic considerations laying out the conceptual approach, study procedures, and the principal dimensions of the Council; (2) a section presenting an analysis of the operation of the mechanism; (3) a final section evaluating the Council and setting forth the conclusions and hypotheses developed from the study.

The conceptual approach and underlying premises of the study, including their relation to relevant writings of other authors, and the research procedures are presented in Chapter 1. The principal dimensions of the Council and its environmental setting, including the main characteristics of the rehabilitation area, are briefly outlined in Chapter 2 in order to acquaint the reader sufficiently with the instrumentality so that he can follow the subsequent analyses. Chapter 3 shows how the Council handled conflict among its members, the conditions under which the members cooperated, and the principal functions that the Council performed for its members. In Chapter 4, the way in which differences in the characteristics of the member agencies affected their calculation of the benefits and costs of cooperation and the rationality of the agencies' behavior in pursuing their self-interests are considered. Chapter 5 discusses the informal rules of the game

individual behavior. Organization theory attempts to account for order in behavior. . . . Organization theory is only concerned with those aspects of behavior which are determined by organizational structures." Thompson goes on to explain "this exclusion of personality . . . may seem wrong to many persons in supervisory positions. Many may feel that most of their problems stem from individual idiosyncracies. They feel this way because they take the organization for granted. The few 'personality cases' are easy to see, and they take up time. The enormous system of order, the organization, goes unnoticed." See *Modern Organization* (New York, 1961), pp. 8–9.

that emerged, the strategies employed by the agencies in advancing and defending their interests, and the processes by which the members interacted in the Council. Chapter 6 examines how the principal actors in the Council's external environment, mainly governors, influenced the mechanism, how they viewed the Council, and what consequences it had for them. Differences in interagency behavior by level, particularly the operation of the regional interdepartmental rehabilitation committees, are the subject of Chapter 7. The problem of evaluating the effectiveness of the Council is considered in Chapter 8, and the performance of the Council is assessed according to various criteria. And last, in Chapter 9 the conclusions and hypotheses that can be drawn from the study are discussed, including the question of what alternatives there are to the Council concept.

Part I

BASIC CONSIDERATIONS

CHAPTER 1

What a Coordinating Council Can Do in Principle

TO answer the question posed by the title of this chapter requires that coordination by council be distinguished from other kinds of coordination and that the principal variables that influence how coordinating councils operate be explained.[1]

Coordination is a vague term that describes most organized effort, for, in its broadest sense, to coordinate is to concert the behavior of interdependent individuals and groups for a particular purpose or end. Consequently, as Philip Selznick has observed, coordination is a term whose meaning must be derived from "the procedures which are established for its effectuation."[2] The concern in this study is with "managed" coordination, which is accomplished by deliberately organized instrumentalities, such as coordinating councils and central budget offices, of which the principal types are coordination by council and coordination by hierarchy.[3] Managed coordination is distinguished from "unman-

1. "Any empirical study must reflect the criteria, implicit or explicit, by which it is decided what data are relevant and what are not." Edward C. Banfield, *Political Influence* (New York, 1961), p. 4.

2. Philip Selznick, *TVA and The Grass Roots* (Berkeley, 1953), p. 64.

3. The coordination of separate organizations (interorganizational) may be distinguished from coordination of the units of a single organization (intraorganizational). Although both types are the same in principle, in

aged" coordination, which occurs in a random or self-regulating fashion, as in a marketplace.[4]

Coordinating councils are much more limited in the degree of coordination they can achieve than hierarchical organizations because they possess much poorer means of controlling their members' behavior. Primarily, coordinating councils, which are peer groups, lack formal authority over their members, and they usually also lack the customary resources, such as funds, manpower, and prestige—resources used by organizations to manipulate their members. By contrast, hierarchical organizations, which are characterized by pyramidal superior-subordinate relations among their members, depend heavily upon formal authority and, equally important, upon dispensing and withholding funds, promotions, and other powerful rewards and punishments to control their members' behavior. Since the members of a coordinating council are coequals organizationally, the group as a whole controls itself, whereas in a hierarchy, control is exerted through a chain of command. The control that coordinating councils have over their members therefore is limited largely to the benefits that the members derive from voluntarily cooperating with each other. Such sanctions as they may be said to possess are the bene-

reality there is likely to be greater control in the latter case, whether the coordination be by council or by hierarchy, for interorganizational coordination is likely to involve fairly autonomous organizations. In reality, interorganizational and intraorganizational mechanisms also blend into one another along a continuum. For example, the degree of autonomy that government departments may have within an executive branch may be comparable to the state of affairs among the units of a holding company.

4. Michael Polanyi argues that science is self-coordinating: "The coordination principle of science consists in the adjustment of each scientist's activities to the results hitherto achieved by others, a basic principle leading generally to coordination without the intervention of any coordinating authority." See *The Logic of Liberty* (Chicago, 1951), pp. 34–35. Charles E. Lindblom advances the thesis that much coordination takes place within and among organizations by means of what he calls processes of "mutual adjustment" (deferring to another, negotiation, bargaining, partisan discussion, etc.). We shall have more to say about this in the last chapter. See *The Intelligence of Democracy* (New York, 1965).

fits that the members may lose from failing to cooperate and the ill will that any member may incur as a result of being uncooperative. Consequently, a coordinating council can act, on its own, and thus coordinate, only on matters on which its members can agree voluntarily. A hierarchical organization, on the other hand, often can induce its members to act in a manner contrary to their preferences.

The advantages of coordination by hierarchy, however, should not be overestimated: such coordination is often difficult to achieve because the means of control upon which it depends have serious weaknesses and unanticipated dysfunctions. For instance, delegating authority to subordinates not only contributes to achievement of organizational goals but also to the emergence of parochial points of view, vested interests, and conflict among the organization's subunits, which tend to subvert the organization's goals.[5] The ability of hierarchical organizations to control the behavior of their personnel by issuing rules and regulations sometimes has undesirable consequences, for rules have a tendency over time to become regarded by those who apply them as ends in themselves, thereby creating internal rigidities and tensions between the organization and its clientele.[6] Similarly, although hierarchical differentiation "is necessary for coordination, it blocks the communication processes that are vital for stimulating initiative and facilitating decision-making."[7] In addition, it usually is very difficult for superiors to tell whether the organization's goals are being realized, for organizational performance is notoriously difficult to measure. It even has been maintained that the merit system of organizational advancement has a tendency to reward self-serving persons at the expense of the organization.[8]

5. Selznick.

6. Robert K. Merton, *Social Theory and Social Structure* (rev. ed.; New York, 1957), pp. 195–206.

7. Peter M. Blau and W. Richard Scott, *Formal Organizations* (San Francisco, 1962), p. 139.

8. Gordon Tullock, *The Politics of Bureaucracy* (Washington, D.C., 1965).

The Conceptual Scheme

This study is about a coordinating council in which certain New York State agencies were required to participate. There was a general expectation that as a body responsible to the governor, the Council would accomplish some coordination. In order therefore to explain how the Council operated, it is essential to identify the principal factors that influenced its performance, of which the most important were certain characteristics of the member agencies and the Council itself.

The agencies belonging to the Council had certain common characteristics as organizations in that they sought to maintain and enhance themselves. They also had the special additional characteristic of being interdependent, for in being members of the executive branch of the state, they shared the same political and administrative environment and performed related health functions.

Organizations generally strive to maintain and enhance themselves, and must if they are to accomplish anything.[9] However, in order to do so, organizations must have purposes that are accepted as legitimate by the larger social system of which they

9. George C. Homans says: "If we are looking at the characteristics that all organizations have in common, we shall do well to speak of the survival motive rather than the profit motive." Also: "The problem . . . is not merely one of survival but also one of the level at which the organization is going to survive. Many organizations try both to survive and to achieve the conditions that will make them better able to survive in the future." See *The Human Group* (New York, 1950), p. 403. Some other representative views are: "But prestige and survival, even for the smallest unit . . . are real factors in decision, as all participants know. Lacking formal channels, necessarily concerned with more than a substantive program, management requires discretion as a means of introducing the factors of prestige and survival into its choices among alternative methods for the execution of formal policy." Selznick, p. 65. "Power relationships are inherent in every administrative situation. The executive must be fully aware of their necessary implications and prepared to struggle openly for power and for survival lest, by false modesty, weakness or self-delusion, he lose or seriously restrict his jurisdiction and endanger his program." Marshall E. Dimock, "Expanding Jurisdictions: A Case Study in Bureaucratic Conflict," in *Reader in Bureaucracy*, ed. Robert K. Merton et al. (New York, 1952), p. 290.

are a part, and they must have access to the resources required to accomplish their objectives, such as funds, manpower, and clients. But legitimated functions and needed resources are in short supply and usually must be obtained from other organizations—a governor or legislature, for example. Typically, there is strong competition for them. Organizations, therefore, generally will defend themselves vigorously against threats to their responsibilities and source of resources and will seize opportunities to expand their purposes and increase their supply of resources.

The maintenance and enhancement needs of organizations are advanced by organization members, since, of course, organizations act through people. When organizations participate in coordinating councils, those who represent them must consider the implications of their actions for their agency's success. Yet, though all personnel are expected to consider their agency's interests (purposes, funds, status, etc.) in dealing with the representatives of other organizations, maintenance of the organization is the primary function of the executive and of his lieutenants. As Clark and Wilson point out:

> Generally, the minimal expectation of group members is that the executive will not allow his group to decline or collapse. The executive's reputation, and in some cases his livelihood and material success, depends upon successful fulfillment of this minimal function. And as many writers have observed, both executives and other contributors come to believe that their organizations must persist if they are to achieve their substantive purposes. Whatever else he may be able to do with or for his group, the executive must perpetuate it.[10]

Thus, in dealing with the behavior of the agencies in the Council, this study focuses upon the actions of its officials as they

10. Peter B. Clark and James Q. Wilson, "Incentive Systems: A Theory of Organization," *Administrative Science Qtly.*, VI (Sept. 1961), 134. Mason Haire reflects: "It seems strange to me that the function of holding the organization together is not more heavily weighted in the job descriptions of executives . . . it seems to me that most time and effort is spent in holding the thing together as a single working unit." See "Biological Models and Empirical Histories of the Growth of Organizations," in *Modern Organization Theory,* ed. Mason Haire (New York, 1959), pp. 302–03.

carried out their functions of maintaining and enhancing their agencies. Since the member agencies were represented in the Council by their chief executives and top officials, except at the regional committee level (rehabilitation), this study mainly is concerned with their behavior as organization members.

The members of a coordinating council are interdependent in that they must "take each other [including the actions of third parties with whom they interact] into account if they are to accomplish their goals."[11] For instance, in the case of the Council, a change by one agency of the standards of eligibility for its services might have affected the number of referrals to another, or one agency might have gained new responsibilities desired by another through action of the legislature.[12]

The response of organizations to interdependence takes two fundamental forms, conflict and cooperation.[13] There is conflict among interdependent organizations when they seek the same functions and resources.[14] On the other hand, such organizations

11. Eugene Litwak and Lydia F. Hylton, "Interorganizational Analysis: A Hypothesis on Coordinating Agencies," *Administrative Science Qtly.*, VI (March 1962), 401.

12. The interdependence of the agencies on any particular matter can be distinguished analytically by whether they are directly dependent upon each other or by whether they are mutually dependent upon a third party. However, on many matters, both types of interdependence are likely to exist.

13. Following the lead of ecologists, Blau and Scott say that the relations among organizations are characterized by two types of processes: competition between like structures for the scarce resources needed for survival and growth; and exchange relations among unlike structures resulting from mutual advantage and dependence. They suggest that competition among formal organizations tends to lead to exchange relations because competition is likely to result in the dominance of some organizations, and they hypothesize that the expandability of formal organizations constitutes a basic limit on this process. The authors also point out that exchange relations may be the obverse of competition: "Social competition, whether between organizations or persons, always involves some kind of exchange relations with other organizations or persons." See Blau and Scott, pp. 214–21.

14. Lewis A. Coser defines social conflict as "a struggle over values and claims to scarce status, power and resources in which the aims of the opponents are to neutralize, injure, or eliminate their rivals." See *The Functions of Social Conflict* (New York, 1956), p. 8. James G. March and Herbert A. Simon, suggest that intergroup conflict is a function of three

are likely to cooperate when they have convergent interests, such as when they are faced with a common threat or can carry out their programs more effectively by taking joint action.[15] Of course, in any given situation, they may not recognize their dependence upon each other and thus neither compete nor cooperate.[16] There also may be considerable variation in the extent to which organizations are interdependent.

Agencies participating in coordinating councils are likely to have both conflicting and convergent interests and thus engage in both competitive and cooperative behavior (outside of the council). Consequently, because of the significance of conflict among organizations, how coordinating councils handle differences among their members and under what conditions their

variables: "The existence of a positive felt need for joint decision-making and of either a difference in goals or a difference in perceptions of reality or both. . . ." See *Organizations* (New York, 1958), p. 121.

15. Sol Levine and Paul E. White present a concept of exchange to explain interorganizational relationships that focuses upon cooperative relationships. Defining exchange as "any voluntary activity between two organizations which has consequences . . . for the realization of their respective goals or objectives," the authors suggest that organizations enter into exchange relationships to obtain clients, labor services, and other resources. Exchange "is contingent upon three related factors: (1) the accessibility of each organization to necessary elements [resources] outside the . . . system [of interrelated organizations], (2) the objectives of the organization and particular functions to which it allocates the elements it controls [which determines the particular elements it needs], and (3) the degree to which domain consensus [agreement on specific goals and functions] exists among the various organizations." With respect to the latter factor the authors say, "Within the . . . system [health agency system in their case], consensus regarding an organization's domain must exist to the extent that parts of the system will provide each agency with the elements necessary to attain its ends." Although their framework does not spell out the kinds of relations that occur among organizations in the absence of these conditions, the view is implicit that organizations will not cooperate or may compete. See "Exchange as a Conceptual Framework for the Study of Interorganizational Relationships," *Administrative Science Qtly.*, V (March 1961), 583–601.

16. This raises the question of the rationality of organizations, which is discussed in Chap. 4. In general, in this study, organizations are assumed to have a high degree of rationality in recognizing and acting on their interests.

members cooperate are among the most important things to know about them.[17]

The members of the council, as line agencies of the executive branch in New York, were no exceptions. They had overlapping health responsibilities and shared a common environment, including the governor, the legislature, and many of the same interest groups. Their interdependence was such that they competed for many of the same resources and cooperated in various ways to fulfill their objectives.

The Council had in common with many other coordinating councils characteristics that significantly affected its operation. Principally, these were somewhat vague purposes, lack of formal authority over its members, and sensitivity to its external environment.

As a formal organizational mechanism, a coordinating council has stated purposes, usually general and vague. Also it is likely to perform informal functions, manifest and latent,[18] for its members and for other groups that have a stake in it. The very generality of its objectives suggests that the informal functions may be particularly important. For instance, some community health councils create the impression that they accomplish more planning than they actually do, and thereby relieve their members of external pressures to integrate their programs. In examining a coordinating

17. In speaking of coordination among organizations, where "there is both conflict and co-operation and formal authority structure is lacking," Litwak and Hylton put the question this way: "What procedures ensure the individual organizations their autonomy in areas of conflict while at the same time permitting their united action in areas of agreement?" They view coordinating agencies, which they define as "formal organizations whose major purpose is to order behavior between two or more other organizations," as a response to these exigencies. This study may be regarded as a partial test of their hypothesis: "Co-ordinating agencies will develop and continue in existence if formal organizations are partly interdependent; agencies are aware of this interdependence, and it can be defined in standardized units of action [requests for funds, information on whether a client is served by another agency, etc.]." See Litwak and Hylton, pp. 396–420.

18. Latent functions are unintended and unrecognized functions, in contradistinction to manifest, or intended, functions. See Merton, *Social Theory and Social Structure*, pp. 19–84.

council, it is therefore essential to look at the functions that it may perform for its members and others. And since a council is a purposive structure, it is, of course, important to consider how well it accomplishes its expressed purposes, as well as any informal functions it may have.

A coordinating council cannot give orders to the member agencies and expect that they will be obeyed. It lacks formal authority, in that the member agencies do not feel an obligation to accept its decisions. The Council had no formally acknowledged rights over the member agencies (such as are conferred by law),[19] and therefore was deficient in one of the most fundamental attributes by which organizations control their members.[20] As a result, coordinating councils are usually unable to dispense the rewards and impose the sanctions that customarily go along with hierarchical position and formal authority—funds, manpower, and status—which organizations also rely upon to gain compliance from their members. Consequently, member agencies within councils may act with considerable autonomy in pursuing their interests. However, coordinating councils necessarily possess some degree of influence over their members, or they could not exist at all. For instance, there must be group norms, or rules of the game, that the

19. Following Banfield, we define authority as influence ("ability to get others to act, think, or feel as one intends") "which rests upon a sense of obligation." See Banfield, p. 4. We also limit it to the sense of obligation felt toward organizational members in superordinate positions. As Robert Presthus points out: "Authority usually rests upon some official position. Although it has several bases of validation, authority is typically legitimated by formal, hierarchical position." See *The Organizational Society* (New York, 1965), p. 136. Commenting upon Max Weber's approach to authority, Blau and Scott set forth three criteria of authority, which amplify our definition: compliance with legitimate commands; suspension of judgment in advance of command; and a value orientation that arises from the group that defines the exercise of social control as legitimate. See Blau and Scott, pp. 27–32.

20. As March and Simon point out: "Acceptance of authority by the . . . [organizational member] gives the organization a powerful means for influencing him—more powerful than persuasion, and comparable to the evoking processes that call forth a whole program of behavior in response to a stimulus." See March and Simon, p. 90.

members are expected to observe, such as honoring agreements, and there are benefits and costs to the agencies of particular courses of action.[21] Because of the lack of formal authority, such factors are especially important in the operation of coordinating councils and should therefore be given particular attention in an analysis of councils.

The external environment in which a coordinating council operates may affect it profoundly. Outside organizations, groups, and individuals are likely to have played a part in its creation and may influence its operation in several ways. They may define its purposes, influence the choice of business that comes before it, and attempt to determine the outcome of decisions that are made. They, of course, also influence a council indirectly through their interaction with the member agencies. For example, in the Council a member agency could decide to bring up for consideration a problem it might be having with the State Civil Service Department. However, outside organizations significantly influence the operation of a council, *qua* council, in three ways: (1) by affecting the structure of the mechanism (for example, the Council was originally established by Governor Thomas E. Dewey by a directive that announced the purposes and membership of the Council); (2) by exerting pressures upon the council that affect the benefits and costs to the member agencies of particular courses of action on the matters that are taken up (for example, the governor could have asked the Council to consider a particular question and to make recommendations to him); (3) by leaving it alone, and thus enabling the members to run it as they see fit.

The approach taken in this study, as all approaches, necessarily presents an incomplete picture of organizational life. But more important, it also presents a viewpoint that can easily be misunderstood. Some readers may object that it gives the impression that the bureaucrats in question are calculating men interested only in aggrandizing their agencies. In focusing upon the behavior

21. For a full treatment of the development and functions of norms in groups, see Homans, *The Human Group,* esp. pp. 121–27.

of New York officials in defending and advancing their agencies' interests, the study deliberately leaves out of consideration the relationships between the officials' actions and their responsibilities to the public, either as they or anyone else saw them. However, in taking this approach, there is no implication that the organization members were interested only in the welfare of their agencies and that they acted only to aggrandize them. Like most public officials, they desired to serve the public well and strove to do so.[22]

More to the point, officials maintain their agencies principally by meeting public needs, for it is largely in this way that they obtain the support that their agencies need to survive. In doing so they and other organization members also obtain such nonmaterial satisfactions as performing their duty, helping others, and being engaged in meaningful work, as well as receiving material rewards. There is necessarily a close relationship between an organization's needs and the interests of those it serves; otherwise it could not survive. As Banfield has observed:

> The maintenance and enhancement needs of a large formal organization . . . can seldom be well served, and often cannot be served at all, by tactics which aim narrowly at the aggrandizement of the organization or which cynically disregard the interest of a larger public. Large formal organizations must offer their contributors (employees, members, customers, etc.) non-material incentives, like the opportunity to be of service to the community or to perform what Barnard has called "ideal benefactions." Thus, paradoxically, the maintenance and enhancement needs of the organization can often only be served by showing that more than mere maintenance or enhancement is being aimed at. By taking a position which its contributors feel is in the public interest, the organization helps to earn their service and loyalty. If it takes a position contrary to what they feel is in the public interest,

22. Recent research suggests that most public officials perceive their agencies "as serving particular groups, as opposed to the general public." See Robert S. Friedman, Bernard W. Klein, and John H. Romani, "Administrative Agencies and the Publics They Serve," *Public Administration Rev.*, XXVI (Sept. 1966), 192–204.

it must offer them some other inducements to make up for the deficiency. Frequently, no others will suffice.[23]

Given its unique characteristics (purposes, traditions, staff composition, etc.) and particular dependence on others (governor, legislature, clientele, etc.), an organization develops a view of how it can best serve others in a way that reflects its maintenance and enhancement needs, which its members may pursue with the conviction and satisfaction that they and their organization are fulfilling their responsibilities. For example, the National Foundation for Infantile Paralysis, now the National Foundation, after virtually accomplishing its original purpose of eradicating poliomyelitis chose, rather than to go out of existence, to take on new responsibilities (arthritis and birth defects) that its members thought were socially desirable and capable of support.[24] The Foundation survived because it was able to convince others (contributors, professional staff, clients, etc.) that they should support its new objectives and thus provide it with the resources needed to pursue its goals rather than turn them over to others. Although some have disagreed with the Foundation's decision, there is no question that generally its members and supporters believe that the organization is fulfilling important health functions.

Similarly, the agencies participating in the Council developed their particular views of the public interest, and in terms of these views they competed and cooperated with each other to serve the public as they saw fit, and in so doing thereby to maintain themselves. They alternately collaborated and vied with each other for the support of such sources of functions and resources as the governor, legislature, and constituent groups. Consequently, they engaged in politics in a broad sense, which they had to do in order to accomplish anything.[25] They would have declined otherwise. As

23. Banfield, p. 264.

24. David L. Sills, *The Volunteers* (New York, 1957).

25. There is, of course, political behavior within organizations too. Peter B. Clark suggests that in a business organization "substantive decisions—decisions which guide actual business operations—are made by processes

one of the Council participants put it, "Any agency worth its salt will fight for what it believes in." But like other organizations the Council agencies varied in the vigor and skill with which they pursued their version of the public interest, and thus in their success.

Although an organization usually must serve others to survive and must persist in order to serve, there may of course be conflict between the maintenance needs of the organization and the interests of the people it serves. For example, in pursuing its maintenance and enhancement needs an agency may resist transfer of some of its functions to another that can better perform them. This study is based upon the premise that the maintenance and enhancement needs of organizations are a fundamental factor governing the behavior of organizations in their relations with other organizations, and that these needs take precedence over other considerations when there is conflict.[26] Furthermore, it is held that this factor determined the extent to which the agencies were able to cooperate in the Council and thus to coordinate their activities.

The Methods of the Study

Customary methods of data collection, including interviews, direct observation, and review of records and other written mate-

which require rather widespread consent," in contrast to "personnel decisions—those dealing with employees' careers, compensation, assignments, and futures—[which] are made by processes which are relatively unilateral and hierarchical." Clark indicates that "the internal 'politics' of the corporation are largely produced by the logical and psychological contradictions which arise between these two decision making procedures." See "The Business Corporation as a Political Order," paper delivered at the 1961 Annual Meeting of the American Political Science Association, St. Louis, Missouri, September 7–9, 1961 (mimeo.).

26. In an interesting study, Walter B. Miller shows how conflicting maintenance needs of diverse community agencies in Boston (courts, religious groups, police, psychiatric agencies, etc.) led to the breakdown of a much-heralded joint community project to prevent juvenile delinquency. See "Inter-Institutional Conflict as a Major Impediment to Delinquency Prevention," *Human Organization,* XVII (Fall 1958), 20–23.

rials, were employed. Approximately 110 persons familiar with the Council were interviewed at length, and often several times, including state officials, present and retired, and private citizens. In all, about 175 interviews were held. The government personnel interviewed consisted of members of the governor's personal staff, the Division of the Budget, the Civil Service Department, the departments participating in the Council (including central office and regional field personnel), the staff of the Council, and the legislature (including legislators and staff). Among the private citizens interviewed were members of state advisory committees, persons influential in the health field in New York, local community health leaders familiar with the Council's regional rehabilitation committees, and others. To facilitate a free flow of information and views, most of the interviews were relatively unstructured. However, several basic questions were asked of most departmental respondents, such as how the Council had been helpful and harmful to their agency and how their agency had perceived the mechanism. Such questions, which were not asked with the intent of tabulating the replies, usually were phrased in different ways in order to probe for similarities and differences of experience and views. Many questions also were posed to check facts and to ascertain the consistency of replies.

For a two-and-a-half-year period, the author had access to all of the meetings of the Council and its committees, including the regional rehabilitation committees. During this time, the operation of the Council was observed at 25 meetings, of which 12 were Council meetings and 13 were committee meetings, mainly on rehabilitation. Direct observation provided an opportunity to get the "feel" of the mechanism and of the style of behavior of the member agencies and their representatives. This was invaluable in gaining insights into the functioning of the Council and in interpreting interviews and written materials. It also was especially helpful in distinguishing between organizational factors and the personality differences that inevitably affect the behavior of departmental representatives in playing their roles as organization members. Furthermore, attendance at meetings made it possible to follow the handling of specific issues, some from start to finish.

Considerable effort was expended in reviewing records, many of which, fortunately, were excellent. All records of the Council over its two-decade history, including agenda, minutes, and related documents, were studied. Their completeness and the unusual care with which they were prepared and preserved greatly facilitated study of the Council's operation. They provided good documentation of the handling of agenda items, supplied many clues to important events and points of view that were pursued in interviews and in other records, and offered a cross check on many facets of Council operation reported on by respondents. These excellent records provided a basis, with further checking, for classifying and tabulating some of the characteristics of all of the rehabilitation issues handled by the Council subsequent to the establishment of its Committee on Rehabilitation in 1953.[27] Records of individual agencies relating to the Council also were made available and, wherever necessary, were examined. And finally, pertinent historical materials were reviewed, such as the papers of the governors, which were available from several sources, particularly the state library.

27. The procedures followed in classifying these issues are described in the Appendix.

CHAPTER 2

Main Dimensions of the Council and Its Setting

THE Council was established in 1946 by executive action of Governor Thomas E. Dewey.[1] Created for the express purpose of providing a "means for assuring cooperation and interchange of plans within the State administration," to assure "coordination of services to people in the local communit[ies],"[2] it brought together the state commissioners of health, mental hygiene, social welfare, and education. In announcing his decision, the Governor said, "The need for such a council is clear. Public Health is a broad field touching many phases of community life. The functions of numerous State agencies in addition to the Department of Health are involved."[3]

The Council took its first breath in a gubernatorial climate that was exceedingly hospitable to such instrumentalities. Much of

1. "Statement—Appointment of Interdepartmental Health Council, October 5, 1946," *Public Papers of Governor Thomas E. Dewey, 1946* (Albany, N. Y., n.d.), pp. 614–15. Contrary to the opinion of some and to the Governor's Press Release of Sept. 23, 1953, announcing enlargement of the Council, an executive order was not issued. For the Council's historical antecedents see Adah Dorothy Bobilin, "The New York Interdepartmental Health Council," unpublished Master's thesis, Syracuse University, 1954, pp. 15–26.

2. "Statement—Appointment of Interdepartmental Health Council, October 5, 1946," p. 615.

3. *Ibid.*, p. 614.

the Dewey administration's interest in the mechanism was based upon a genuine conviction that interdepartmental committees are useful coordinating devices. Such bodies were very popular at that time, and in the words of a former state official who had many different assignments in the administration, "Dewey was very well satisfied and thought they were very effective. . . . They were subscribed to so heavily . . . [that] they were a burden to the commissioners."

The administration's public image, however, was the precipitating factor in establishing the mechanism. In fact, the Council was born of an awkward situation in which the Governor had to make a dramatic move in the health field. As World War II drew to a close, pressures for compulsory health insurance were reasserted in New York. Thus, on Governor Dewey's recommendation, the legislature, in 1944, established a distinguished Commission on Medical Care "to make necessary studies, in order to devise programs of medical care for persons of all age groups and classes."[4] But the Commission turned out to be a public fiasco, as its 18 members split into five factions, each of which issued its own report. Even the majority report was subscribed to by only half of the members.

Forewarned and concerned, the Governor moved to pick up the pieces before the Commission officially reported to him. He quickly called together a group of top aides and advisors, whom he asked to come up with a prompt answer to the question: "What is there we can do in public health?" as one aide put it. The committee, which was called the Governor's Informal Committee on Public Health, lost no time in responding to the Governor's charge. In several weeks it put together a comprehensive program to expand public health services, including a proposal to create an Interdepartmental Health Council. Nine days later, and shortly after the ill-fated Commission report was issued, Governor Dewey submitted the Committee's recommendations to the legislature

4. *Medical Care for the People of New York* (Albany, N. Y., Feb. 15, 1946), p. 1.

in a special message in which he announced his intention to set up the Council as part of the package. It was evident to most observers that the Governor's recommendations were a substitute for what the Commission failed to produce:

> There has already been submitted to your Honorable Bodies the five separate reports of the members of the Commission on Medical Care which reflect the sharp disagreement amongst all people as to the means by which a broad program for medical care can be provided. Obviously, this problem must await further study and disposition by the Congress of bills on this subject pending before it.
>
> In the field of public health I have the pleasure and honor to present to you a definite and comprehensive program for the benefit of our people which is free from confusion and which I am sure will not entail disagreement as to its broad principles.[5]

The proposal to create the Council originated with two members of the Governor's Informal Committee, which was chaired by the Commissioner of Health. One was Assemblyman Lee Mailler, who for years had headed a distinguished legislative commission that since 1939 repeatedly had recommended establishment of "a representative interdepartmental council on a State level to guide health activities in the various State departments."[6] Mailler also was a trusted advisor of the Governor. The other was Doctor John J. Bourke, Secretary of the Joint Hospital Board, who, assisted by an aide of the Director of the Budget, drafted the report of the Committee. Bourke, a public health officer by profession, had been research director of the "Mailler Commission" while on loan from the Department of Health. In this capacity he had helped prepare the Commission's recommendations for an Interdepartmental Health Council. When the idea was presented to the Governor's Informal Committee, the other members accepted it without dissent but apparently with no special enthu-

5. "Message Submitting a Comprehensive Public Health Program, March 4, 1946," *Public Papers of Governor Thomas E. Dewey, 1946* (Albany, N. Y., n.d.), p. 97.

6. *Medical Care in New York State, 1939*, Legislative Document No. 91 (Albany, N. Y., 1940), p. 9.

siasm as well. The Governor later paid tribute to Mailler's and Bourke's influence when he personally suggested that Mailler be a member of the new Council and that Bourke be its part-time secretary. Thus was the Council born of the fortuitous convergence of three factors: Governor Dewey's need to overcome the failure of his Commission on Medical Care; his belief in the value of interdepartmental coordinating devices; and the views on interdepartmental coordination of the Mailler Commission.

Since its creation, the Council was reorganized by two succeeding state administrations and its membership expanded and contracted over the years. Nevertheless, it saw little essential change in two decades. For example, its basic purposes did not vary, generally the same subject areas dominated its interests, and the original four departments constituted a membership core throughout its life. During its IHHC phase, the Council had five departmental members, the original four—Health, Mental Hygiene, Social Welfare, Education—plus Insurance. However, many more agencies were represented on its committees, as is shown later.

Organization and Reorganization

The history of the Council divides into three distinct phases that coincide roughly with changes in state administrations. It is important to distinguish these phases because of the ways in which they have affected the Council's legal basis, purposes, membership, and structure: the first, as the Interdepartmental Health Council (IHC), 1946–1956 (Dewey administration, January, 1943, to December, 1954); the second, as the Interdepartmental Health Resources Board (IHRB), 1956–1960 (Harriman administration, January, 1955, to December, 1958); and its final phase, as the Interdepartmental Health and Hospital Council (IHHC), 1960 to 1967 (Rockefeller administration, January, 1959, to the present).[7]

7. New York governors serve four-year terms.

IHC Phase, 1946–1956

During the Dewey administration the Council's purposes were broad and general. The executive power of the Governor provided the legal foundation for the Council, but beyond determining the Council's composition, the Governor, in a brief directive, neither spelled out its structure nor indicated how it was to operate. With regard to its functions he merely said, "In addition to coordinating activities already undertaken or to be started this year [the Council] will have the function of studying and recommending action on unmet or inadequately covered public health needs."[8] Especially notable was the directive's silence on the question of the Council's legal authority over its members, either regarding implementation of its decisions or concerning its needs for information and staff. None of the subsequent reorganizations have really broken this silence.[9]

The original membership consisted of the four core departments and an advisory member from the legislature, Assemblyman Mailler, who became Assembly Majority leader four months after the Council was created.[10] In 1953 the membership was expanded by a second executive directive, which added the Department of Labor (Industrial Commissioner); the Department of Correction (Commissioner of Correction); the Workmen's Compensation Board of the Department of Labor (Chairman); and the Division of Parole of the Executive Department (Chairman).[11] In

8. "Statement—Appointment of Interdepartmental Health Council, October 5, 1946," p. 615.

9. In a subsequent reorganization (1956), the Council was "authorized to request any department or agency represented on the board [Council] to provide such facilities, including personnel, assistance and data, as will enable the board [Council] properly to carry out its activities," but nothing was said about the members' obligation to comply. See *New York Laws of 1956,* Chap. 191.

10. Mailler had chaired the Temporary Legislative Commission to Formulate a Long Range State Health Program (Health Preparedness Commission), which as early as 1939 had recommended establishment of an interdepartmental council to coordinate health services. See *Medical Care in New York State, 1939,* p. 9.

11. "Appointments, Interdepartmental Health Council, September 22, 1953," *Public Papers of Governor Thomas E. Dewey, 1953* (Albany, N. Y., n.d.), p. 482.

1954 the advisory member withdrew when he resigned from the legislature and was appointed to the chairmanship of the Division of Parole. He was not replaced in his former role because his appointment to the Council had been influenced more by his personal interests and qualifications than by institutional considerations.

Throughout the IHC phase the Commissioner of Health was permanent chairman of the Council. Although the originating directive was silent on this point, it was informally understood that the Commissioner of Health would chair the Council. From the beginning it was felt that the Department of Health had the greatest stake in Council affairs. However, this was much less true during the subsequent phases, when the chairman was elected annually and the custom of rotating the office was observed. The Dewey administration also did not make any provision for funds or staff, leaving this up to the members. During this period Dr. John J. Bourke, the executive director of the Joint Hospital Survey and Planning Commission, itself an independent interdepartmental agency, staffed the Council and its committees with assistance from his aides and the member agencies.[12]

Generally the Council was concerned with long-standing problems of interest to its members, though it also was sensitive to the changing character and priority of problems. Thus the pattern of interests that emerged during the first decade continued throughout the life of the Council. Although some problems and some priorities changed, the main problems that continued to engage the Council were: rehabilitation, nursing, alcoholism, narcotics addiction, health manpower, and medical care and hos-

12. The Joint Hospital Survey and Planning Commission, originally known as the Joint Hospital Board of the Postwar Public Works Planning Commission, until it was established as a separate entity by the legislature in 1947, was the state's mechanism for carrying out the provisions of the Federal Hospital Survey and Construction Act (Hill-Burton). It was composed of the Commissioners of Health, Mental Hygiene, and Social Welfare. It was abolished in 1960 and most of its functions transferred to the Department of Health. For the early history of the Commission, see Lynton K. Caldwell, *The Government and Administration of New York*, American Commonwealth Series (New York, 1954), pp. 357–58.

pitals. School health is the only area once of major concern in this period that eventually became dormant. Several problems also came to the fore subsequent to the IHC period, mainly mental retardation, emotionally disturbed children, and aging.

IHRB Phase, 1956–1960

The Harriman administration also thought well of the Council and even outdid its predecessor in supporting it. On the administration's recommendation, the Council was raised to the status of an independent agency and its membership and functions were broadened.[13] The enabling act, which spanned four years, affirmed the Council's original purpose: "To make possible joint and mutual planning and action by several state departments and boards in regard to health and mental health problems of the people of the state," and it spelled out these additional functions: "To initiate, formulate, . . . execute and transfer as soon as feasible to appropriate permanent state administrative agencies programs," including but not limited to alcoholism, mental retardation, emotionally disturbed children, rehabilitation, and aging.[14] Although the law used the terms "power" and "duty" in assigning these functions, it did not actually increase the legal authority of the Council vis-à-vis its members. It did expand the functions of the Council to permit initiation and operation of some research and demonstration programs with the qualification that eventually they would be assigned to a permanent operating agency. Immediately upon its reorganization, the Council was assigned several projects in the fields of alcoholism, mental retardation, and emotionally disturbed children that were carried over from the Mental Health Commission, an expiring temporary interdepartmental commis-

13. "Message Concerning Public Health and Mental Health, January 17, 1956," *Public Papers of Governor W. Averell Harriman, 1956* (Albany, N. Y., n.d.), pp. 49–50.

14. *New York Laws of 1956,* Chap. 191. Legally, the Council was a temporary agency, as the New York Constitution, then as now, limits the number of civil departments. See *New York Constitution, 1938,* as amended, Art. 5, Secs. 2 and 3.

sion.[15] Taking over these projects was the closest the Council ever came to being an operating agency. The enabling act and a subsequent amendment also increased the Council's membership to include the Joint Hospital Survey and Planning Commission (Executive Director) and the Youth Commission (Chairman).[16]

The Council reached the high point of its formality and visibility during the IHRB period. As an independent agency responsible directly to the governor, it acquired an executive head (executive director), a budget, and a modest full-time staff. The law also called for the annual election of the chairman, which led to the tradition of rotating the chairmanship among the four core departments. Written bylaws interpreting Council functions and spelling out policies and operating procedures also were adopted. These strengthened the hand of the executive director, particularly by making him chairman ex officio of all Council committees. Thus the previous custom of choosing departmental representatives as committee chairman was overturned, only, however, to be reinstituted in the IHHC period. Also for the first time, advisory committees, which coopted representatives of private groups, were organized in the fields of alcoholism and mental retardation.[17] These were a carry-over from the Mental Health Commission. Moreover, annual reports were prepared, as provided for by law.

15. The Interdepartmental Health Resources Board was created in effect by combining the functions of the Interdepartmental Health Council and some of the functions of the Mental Health Commission, which had been established by the legislature in 1949 to develop a master plan for the promotion of mental health programs. Composed of the Commissioners of Health, Mental Hygiene, Social Welfare, Education, and Correction, the Commission had begun several projects of interdepartmental interest that were transferred to the reformed Council. Their transfer increased the Council's interest in mental health. For origins of the Mental Health Commission, see Caldwell, pp. 355–57.

16. *New York Laws of 1956*, Chap. 191, and *New York Laws of 1959*, Chap. 249, respectively.

17. Philip Selznick defines cooptation as "the process of absorbing new elements into the leadership or policy-determining structure of an organization as a means of averting threats to its stability or existence." It may be done formally or informally. See *TVA and The Grass Roots* (Berkeley, 1949), p. 13.

IHHC Phase, 1960–1967

The Council experienced its most severe reorganization early in the Rockefeller administration, when the legislation establishing the IHRB was allowed to expire in implementation of the Governor's plan for reorganizing the executive branch.[18] Probably the Council would have been abolished had not the commissioners of the four core departments, under the leadership of the Commissioner of Health, sought to save the mechanism, for at the time the administration considered the Council a liability. The final form of the Council, which was created by executive order,[19] represented a compromise with the Rockefeller administration, which, though its views mellowed with time, had little interest in supporting the mechanism. In this reorganization, the Council was stripped of the operating functions gained during the Harriman administration, and the six agencies that were the least active participants—Labor, Workmen's Compensation, Correction, Parole, Joint Hospital Survey and Planning Commission, and the Youth Commission—were dropped, and the Department of Insurance was added. Thus the final membership consisted of five.[20]

Although the reorganization lowered the status and visibility of the Council, the Governor's executive order reaffirmed its purpose: To provide a vehicle for the continued exchange of information and for cooperative study and action by the State agencies with responsibilities in the fields of health and hospital care."[21] Moreover, its functions were spelled out more clearly in this order

18. *Proposed Reorganization of the Executive Branch of New York State Government, Report to Governor Nelson A. Rockefeller* (Albany, N. Y., Dec. 1959).

19. "Executive Order Establishing an Interdepartmental Health and Hospital Council, March 31, 1960," *Public Papers of Governor Nelson A. Rockefeller, 1960* (Albany, N. Y., n.d.), pp. 985–86.

20. In the reorganization of the executive branch, the Joint Hospital Survey and Planning Commission and the Youth Commission were abolished; most of the functions of the former were transferred to the Department of Health; the latter agency was made a division of the Executive Department.

21. "Executive Order Establishing an Interdepartmental Health and Hospital Council, March 31, 1960," p. 985.

than in earlier promulgations. Drawing in large measure from the previous bylaws and reflecting actual practice, the order enumerated these functions:

To conduct joint study, planning, and program development . . . To serve as organized medium of exchange of information . . . to develop appropriate approaches or recommendations to the Governor. . . . To establish [a] framework for interdepartmental consultation.[22]

In losing its standing as an independent agency, the Council also formally lost its right to a separate budget and staff. Subsequent to 1960, its staff, which reverted to a secretarial role, was provided for in the budget of the Health Department, and the Department furnished such administrative housekeeping services as were required. It is notable that the Department seems not to have taken advantage of this situation to influence the Council, although some members felt that the arrangement identified the Council too closely with the Department. The staff and funds of the Council also were reduced with the transfer of its pilot research and demonstration programs to the member departments. An executive secretary and a special assistant, who were carried over from the IHRB phase, constituted the sole professional staff.[23]

Mode of Operation

The Council operated by means of regularly scheduled meetings of the commissioners and of committees of their lieutenants, at which information and views were exchanged and some decisions were made. Aided by a formal agenda prepared by the staff and cleared with the chairman, the commissioners—since the early

22. *Ibid.*

23. Several additional professional staff members who had been supervised by Council staff had served on a temporary basis on special projects of direct interest to the Council, but these projects were carried out under the aegis of the Governor's Council on Rehabilitation, a citizen advisory committee. See Chap. 6.

years—met monthly, usually for two or three hours, except during summer months. A remarkable fact was the high level of attendance of the commissioners of the core agencies. From the very first meeting, they agreed to attend meetings themselves, a practice they adhered to with unusual faithfulness. The executive heads of the four core departments, whose agencies had the most to gain or lose through participation, as a group attended almost 80 percent of all the meetings of the Council.[24] These same commissioners also invariably sent representatives in their absence, and some followed the practice of having one of their top aides attend regularly with them. Thus the core agencies as a group were represented at 96 percent of all the meetings.[25]

The frequency of committee meetings was variable. Among the Council's nine committees active during the IHHC phase, the pattern ranged from meetings held monthly to several times a year, with bimonthly a rough average. Here again the general practice was for staff to prepare agenda in consultation with the committee chairman. Attendance at committee meetings also was high, as the core agencies as a whole were represented at 85 percent of the meetings of the seven most active committees during the IHRB and IHHC periods.[26]

Although the meetings of the Council and of most committees followed written agenda, often prepared with impressive supporting documentation, the atmosphere of the meetings was informal and usually relaxed. Only members attended, except guests invited to participate in the discussion of specific topics. It was most unusual for a member of the governor's staff to be present, and until late in the IHHC period it was not customary to send copies of the minutes to the governor and his aides.

24. See Table 2, p. 80.
25. See Table 1, p. 79.
26. Includes the committees on rehabilitation, nursing, mental retardation, emotionally disturbed children, aging, alcoholism, and narcotics addiction during the period between April, 1956, and December, 1964. The core agencies' attendance ranged from 69 percent (narcotics addiction) to 95 percent (nursing).

From the very first meeting, the commissioners organized committees to conduct the bulk of the work of the Council, so that the pattern of committees closely reflected the commissioners' substantive interests. It also was a policy from the outset to invite other agencies to full membership on committees that were concerned with matters involving their interests. Thus, during the final phase, twelve agencies, in addition to the five member departments, participated in one or more active committees.[27] Chairmen of committees were generally elected by the members, usually for one year, except that during the IHRB phase the executive director chaired all the committees.

Except for this period, the role of the Council's staff was primarily secretarial: preparation of agenda, minutes, and reports; assembling of information; and conduct and supervision of special studies. However, since they were professionally qualified and well respected, the incumbents also exercised a fair amount of informal influence, as for example in the choice of agenda items. This influence was at its height during the IHRB period. The former executive director estimated that he suggested about 30 percent of the agenda items of the Council. Staff also represented the Council in negotiations with other agencies and handled most of its communications. Moreover, beginning with the IHRB period, it was customary for staff to report regularly at meetings on the work of the committees and related groups.

The Environmental Setting and the Council Members

The Council operated within a relatively stable governmental structure accustomed to strong executive leadership and to a highly disciplined legislature. Usually the governor and the legis-

27. The twelve are: Department of Agriculture nad Markets; Department of Civil Service; Department of Commerce; Department of Conservation; Department of Correction; the Divisions of Parole, Youth, and Housing and the Office of Aging of the Executive Department; the Division of Employment and the Workmen's Compensation Board of the Department of Labor; and the Department of Public Works.

lature came from the same political party, and chief executives traditionally enjoyed long tenures. "The legislature of the State possesses a party discipline far superior to that found either in the United States congress or in all but a few state capitals. . . . Consequently, the process of legislation consists of a process of negotiation among the legislative leaders of the two houses and the governor."[28] And as another observer has noted, the state also has "one of the tightest patterns of budgetary control in the nation."[29] The Council was therefore relatively insulated from the legislature, for insofar as legislators were conscious of it they regarded it as an executive instrumentality of little direct concern to them.

As one of the wealthiest and most populous states, New York enjoys a position of political and administrative leadership. Its governors almost automatically become presidential contenders,[30] and its programs in the fields of health, education, and welfare are among the largest and most highly developed in the country. Consequently, the agencies belonging to the Council enjoyed national recognition, and their executives and professional staffs were accustomed to playing prominent roles in the professional associations and interest groups active in their fields. As one would expect, they were proud and jealous of such preeminence. Council members were therefore sensitive to trends and developments on the national scene in their areas of interest, many of which they helped to fashion.

Twenty regular departments, limited in number by the Constitution,[31] carry out the major administrative functions of the state,

28. Ralph A. Straetz and Frank J. Munger, *New York Politics* (New York, 1960), p. 61. The impact of the Johnson landslide in 1964, which gave the Democrats undisputed control of both houses for the first time in many years, and of reapportionment, which is diminishing traditional Republican strength, seem to threaten this pattern.

29. Morris Schaefer, "Area and Function in the Administration of Public Health in New York State," unpublished doctoral dissertation, Syracuse University, 1962, p. 355.

30. Straetz and Munger, p. 1.

31. See Note 14, above.

of which thirteen participated in the Council, five as members, and eight more on one or more committees.[32] The combined operations of the five members of the Council for all purposes, in 1965, accounted for 69 percent of the total state budget of more than three billion dollars, or a little over two billion dollars.[33] Ranked in order of magnitude their individual budgets came to approximately: Education, slightly more than a billion dollars; Mental Hygiene, $299 million; Social Welfare, $589 million; Health, $106 million; and Insurance, $8 million.[34] As one would anticipate, the combined budgets of the Council members for health purposes also made up the lion's share of the 20 percent of the State budget roughly estimated to be earmarked for health and health-related purposes.[35]

There are sharp differences in the extent to which each of the departments that were members of the Council performs health functions.[36] The Departments of Health and Mental Hygiene are the state's major health agencies, dividing between them the traditional public health functions, which in some states are the province of a single agency. The Department of Health is responsible for most of the recognized public health functions: control of environmental hazards, such as air and water pollution; control of communicable and chronic diseases, through operation of facilities and programs for such groups as the tuberculous, chroni-

32. In the case of several departments, several of their units are represented on committees. See Note 27, above.

33. Based on figures provided by the Division of the Budget.

34. *Ibid.*

35. Estimated by the author using figures supplied by the Division of the Budget.

36. The ramifications in the state of Social Security Amendments of 1965 ("Medicare"—Public Law 89–97, 89th Cong., H.R. 6675, July 30, 1965) and recent state legislation (particularly *New York Laws of 1965*, Chap. 795, and *New York Laws of 1966*, Chaps. 256, 257, 799–802) are changing many of the agencies' functions and thus their relationships. *New York Laws of 1965* represents a basic change in state policy that occurred independently of Medicare, whereas *New York Laws of 1966* in large measure implements federal policy (Medicare), which is partly inconsistent with previous state policy. The following summarizes the agencies' functions as of the end of 1965, before Medicare and the state laws became effective.

cally ill, and physically handicapped; and more recently, development of standards and programs to assure adequate distribution and quality of medical services, which have been expanded considerably by Medicare and recent state legislation. Most of its activities are carried on through the administration of state aid and by supervision of county and city health departments. The basic function of the Department of Mental Hygiene is care and treatment of the mentally ill and mentally defective. In carrying out this responsibility, the Department operates an extensive system of hospitals, schools, and other facilities, and it administers a relatively new and expanding program of state aid to localities for the development and operation of community mental health services.

Health is a secondary function for the other three departments that were Council members, but they nevertheless have substantial responsibilities. The Department of Social Welfare, which supervises a wide variety of locally administered public welfare programs, was responsible during the period covered by the study for medical assistance for the indigent and medical assistance for the aged, which also have been changed substantially by Medicare and recent state legislation.[37] It was also responsible for the inspection of hospitals, nursing homes, and convalescent homes, many of which are operated by local welfare agencies.[38] The Education Department, which administers the most costly program of state aid to localities (school districts), also has major health functions. They embrace health education of school children and school health services, including school sanitation;[39] education and licensing of physicians and other health professionals; and vocational rehabilitation, which has a large medical

37. Responsibility for the medical aspects of these programs has been transferred to the Department of Health.

38. Legislation enacted in 1965 and effective Feb. 1, 1966, transferred the responsibilities for inspection of hospitals and nursing homes to the Department of Health. See *New York Laws of 1965*, Chap. 795.

39. In a few cities (New York, Buffalo, and Rochester) this function is the responsibility of public health officials.

component. The Department of Insurance is involved in health matters through its responsibilities for the regulation of health insurance. Other departments, most of which were represented on one or more Council committees, also have important health functions, but there is no need to consider them here.

Rehabilitation

Since this study focuses somewhat more upon the Council's operation in the area of rehabilitation than on its other activities, some introductory comments are appropriate.

Although the boundaries of this program sector are vague and blend into other activities, rehabilitation is principally a comprehensive interdisciplinary approach to meeting the multiple needs of handicapped persons.[40] Rehabilitation also is the most widely interdepartmental subject area in which the Council was active. Nine different agencies, each having different but related rehabilitation responsibilities, participated in the Committee on Rehabilitation, more than in any other committee. Consequently, there were differences of opinion among the member agencies over the proper scope of the Committee's concern with the subject. Nevertheless, the members agreed in general terms to limit their interest in rehabilitation to programs: "To overcome the composite problems of disabled individuals, so that they achieve maximal development or restoration of their physical, mental, social and vocational capacities for self-sufficiency, social adjustment and employment."[41]

In practice, however, the Committee was more concerned with the physically handicapped, including their emotional, social, and vocational needs, than with mentally ill or mentally retarded persons without physical disabilities. Other Council committees

40. Basil J. F. Mott, *Financing and Operating Rehabilitation Centers and Facilities* (Chicago, 1960), pp. 9–16.

41. *New York State Programs in Rehabilitation, A Report by the Board Committee on Rehabilitation, to the Interdepartmental Health Resources Board* (Albany, N. Y., Dec. 1, 1959), p. 6.

dealt with the latter groups. The Committee on Rehabilitation also specifically excluded from its jurisdiction groups requiring social rehabilitation, such as probationers and parolees, except those "with physical, mental, or emotional disabilities who are capable of benefiting from rehabilitation services."[42]

Discounting some earlier activity, the Council's active interest in rehabilitation began in 1953, when, encouraged by the Department of Health, its members established the Committee on Rehabilitation. Although no single event precipitated the formation of the Committee, the principal factors at the time were a growing national interest in rehabilitation and the desire of the Health Department to expand its rehabilitation and medical functions. In the early 1950's, this interest, which gained impetus from the dramatic success in rehabilitating severely disabled servicemen wounded in World War II, was reflected in new and expanding federal programs and growing private activity. The rehabilitation movement, as some have called it, even developed something of a missionary fervor, which it still possesses to some degree.

In addition to having the longest continuous history, the Committee on Rehabilitation held more meetings than any other committee (92 in the 12 years since its formation); it met more frequently than other major committees (8.5 times per year during the IHRB period, and 10.4 times per year in the IHHC period); its meetings were among the best attended (88 percent for the core agencies during the IHRB and IHHC periods); and, in the opinion of almost everyone interviewed, it was the most productive group.[43]

As one might expect, the rehabilitation activities of the nine agencies that belonged to the Committee on Rehabilitation are varied as well as often closely related. Furthermore, their diver-

42. Report of the Sub-Committee to Determine the IHHC Rehabilitation Committee Responsibility for Probationers, Parolees, and Prisoners, Feb. 6, 1964. Exhibit III of the Minutes of the Committee on Rehabilitation, Jan. 20, 1964.

43. See Note 26, above. The cut-off date of these computations is Dec. 1964. More current data show that this pattern was continued for the life of the Council.

sity and relationship to other departmental programs shows that they could not be combined in a single department without a major reorganization of other agency functions. To summarize them briefly, covering the period of the study:[44] The Department of Health in conjunction with local communities is responsible for partial funding and approval of medical rehabilitation services to children. It also provides services to adults, for the Department operates a special rehabilitation hospital and tuberculosis sanatoria, and conducts and helps finance various special clinics offering rehabilitation services. Moreover, since 1960, it has administered the federal hospital construction program, which provides funds for rehabilitation facilities,[45] and a state program of continuing financial assistance to rehabilitation centers.[46] The Department of Mental Hygiene, which considers rehabilitation as an objective of the entire department, provides specific rehabilitative services, such as physical and occupational therapy in hospitals for the mentally ill and in schools for the severely mentally retarded. It also supports rehabilitation services through community mental health programs. The Department of Social Welfare helps finance medical rehabilitation services for the medically indigent as well as for persons on public assistance. It also administers the federal-state program of vocational rehabilitation for the blind, which includes medical and other benefits; furthermore, the agency determines the eligibility of persons for disability benefits under the federal program of old-age and survivors' insurance (Social Security). Similarly, the State Education Department has a large stake in rehabilitation. It is responsible for the federal-state program of vocational rehabilitation for all persons other than the blind, which has a significant medical component, and which includes responsibilities for construction and expansion of rehabilitation facilities. The Department also is

44. See Note 36, above.

45. These functions were transferred to the Department of Health from the Joint Hospital Survey and Planning Commission, when the latter agency was abolished in 1960. See Note 12, above.

46. See Chap. 7.

responsible for a fairly new state program of continuing financial assistance to sheltered workshops, which employ and help rehabilitate the handicapped. Moreover, the Department supervises and helps finance a wide range of special educational and therapeutic services provided for handicapped children during their school years. The Employment Service of the Department of Labor operates a selective placement program to assist handicapped persons to find jobs, which is integrated with its basic employment program. The Workmen's Compensation Board, a relatively autonomous unit of the Labor Department, which, for that reason, is treated as a separate agency in this study, also has a rehabilitation program. In processing workers' claims for compensation and medical benefits, the Board actively encourages, and under certain conditions requires, employers and insurance companies to pay for rehabilitation services. The Governor's Committee on Employ the Handicapped, which has a federal counterpart, carries out an educational program to foster employment of disabled persons. Since, for housekeeping purposes, the Committee is in the Department of Labor, it also is considered as a separate agency in this study. The Department of Correction provides some rehabilitation services, mainly of a social character, to its inmate population and to probationers. Although it does not have custodial responsibilities, the Division of Parole furnishes similar services to parolees.

Part II

ANALYSIS OF THE COUNCIL

CHAPTER 3

Conflict and Cooperation

THE most serious obstacles to coordinating the efforts of separate organizations stem from disagreements among them, such as those that arise when organizations have conflicting objectives, or when they compete for the same resources. Consequently, a most significant characteristic of a coordinating council is how it deals with conflict among the agencies it attempts to coordinate. Equally important are the conditions under which the members engage in cooperative behavior.

It will therefore be instructive (1) to show how the Council handled conflict among its members and to describe the conditions under which the agencies cooperated; (2) to identify the advantages and disadvantages of participating in the Council from the members' point of view, and to show how these factors affected operation of the mechanism; and (3) to spell out the principal functions that the Council performed for its members.

The Council was not a mechanism for the direct management of conflict among its members, although it had significant indirect functions in this regard—for example, as a listening post and as a sounding board. Left to the control of its members, as was largely the case, the Council could act only by voluntary agreement—that is, when some of its members gained and none lost. Consequently, Council business seldom involved much conflict, and when substantial disagreement did arise over agenda items, the Council rarely resolved it.[1] Furthermore, the more intense the potential conflict, the less likely it was that an issue would become an agenda item, and if it did, the less likely that it would be resolved. This tendency to avoid controversy, and thus to cooperate only when it was mutually advantageous, was closely related to the structure of the Council and to the benefits and costs of cooperation. As is shown in a later chapter, avoidance of controversy was reflected in the informal rules of the game that governed the members' behavior and in the processes by which the Council operated.[2] In this discussion it is necessary to establish relevant organizational facts; accordingly a brief description follows of the Council's response to high-conflict issues.

Avoiding Conflict

The Council's avoidance of conflict certainly did not result from lack of competition or disagreement among the member agencies. On the contrary, the struggle among the members for functions, resources, and such related intangibles as status and prestige was at times intense, as might be expected of prominent and ambitious agencies.[3] Examination of the main points of friction among the four core agencies reveals that the issues involved rarely were put before the Council and that those that were usually were rejected or not resolved.[4]

Most of the rivalry among the Council agencies involved the Department of Health. As most of the officials interviewed agreed,

1. Agenda items are defined as all matters considered by the Council. They vary from simple exchanges of information to joint decisions on actions to be taken. See Note 17, below.

2. See Chap. 5.

3. See Chap. 1 for a discussion of the organizational premises underlying this study, esp. pp. 18–21.

4. Since the most important conflicts have occurred among the four core members, only these disagreements are discussed in the interests of brevity. The Council behaves no differently, however, with respect to other controversies.

that department pursued its version of the public interest with more vigor and self-assurance than the other agencies, for the Department has always been convinced that it is better qualified to perform certain of the health functions assigned to other agencies. Therefore, the behavior of the Department of Health, as will be shown, particularly affected the operation of the Council.[5] However, each of the core members clashed at least once with another member besides Health. Nine major areas of disagreement, involving either the possible transfer of functions from one department to another or competition for new or developing ones, stand out. These conflict areas are best described by pairs of departments inasmuch as each generally brought into play the interests of two departments at one time. To simplify the discussion only the major interests of the departments are examined.

Conflict between Health and Education. Most of the disagreement between the Departments of Health and Education centered on two issues: namely the desire of the Department of Health to take over from the Education Department state responsibilities for health services to school children, including school sanitation, and responsibility for the medical aspects of the programs of the Division of Vocational Rehabilitation. Although the Department of Health asked the Council early in its history to consider these issues, and also made some headway outside of the Council in persuading the Commissioner of Education of the merits of its case, the issues were shunned by the Council. The issues were nonetheless implicit in many of the deliberations on school health and on rehabilitation, both at the committee level and among the commissioners, and the representatives from each of the departments were well aware of the underlying conflict. Yet, even though the Council reached agreement on some aspects of the problems concerning school health and vocational rehabili-

5. The vigorousness of the Department of Health made the Council an especially good subject for research. Since the Department pushed the Council about as far as possible in seeking to realize its view of the public interest, it accentuated the dynamics of the Council mechanism, especially its capacity to deal with conflict.

tation, there was neither direct confrontation nor resolution of the basic issues.

Conflict between Health and Social Welfare. Two issues produced most of the disagreement between the Department of Health and the Department of Social Welfare: (1) responsibility for the medical aspects of the state's public welfare programs, and (2) responsibility for inspection and regulation of hospitals and nursing homes. The Department of Health considered itself best equipped to perform both of these functions, which traditionally have been the province of the Department of Social Welfare. Feeling very strongly about hospital inspection, which in most states is looked upon as a public health responsibility, the Department of Health fought hard and skillfully, and with success, to develop sufficient support to have this function transferred to its jurisdiction.[6] Neither of these two principal issues was ever brought to the Council, except obliquely, and one instance graphically illustrates the point. In 1962, Governor Rockefeller responded to growing public concern about the high cost of hospital and nursing home care with a message to the legislature that called upon the Council to assist in developing a model nursing-home code.[7] When the message, which the Department of Health welcomed, was considered by the Council, the Commissioner of Social Welfare demurred, pointing out that his department was responsible for the regulation of nursing homes. After some discussion it was decided that the message was unclear and that therefore the Governor's office should be asked for clarification. At that point the matter passed from Council concern, except for subsequent reports by representatives of the Department of Social Welfare of their progress in revising nursing home regulations.

Conflict between Health and Mental Hygiene. Most of the disagreement between the Departments of Health and Mental

6. See Note 38, Chap. 2, p. 38.

7. "Message of Governor Nelson A. Rockefeller to the Legislature, January 3, 1962," Legislative Document No. 1, 1962 (Albany, N. Y., n.d.), pp. 29–30.

Hygiene arose from differences over responsibility for state programs for alcoholics, narcotics addicts, and mentally retarded children. In the case of alcoholism, both departments sought to be designated as the primary agency for what was essentially a new and developing program, whereas in the case of narcotics addiction, one of the parties was reluctant to take on a new and politically thankless responsibility, yet did not want the other to have it.[8]

The alcoholism issue was placed squarely before the Council; nevertheless the question was dropped. During its IHRB phase, the Council inherited responsibility from the Mental Health Commission for the state's fledgling alcoholism program, which consisted of several research and demonstration clinics initiated by the Commission.[9] By law, the Council was required to transfer its pilot programs to a permanent line agency when feasible. Thus, when the question of transferring its programs came up in the closing days of the IHRB, the Council was confronted by a dilemma: it had to decide, between two determined competitors, what to do with its alcoholism program. Both the Department of Health and the Department of Mental Hygiene were firmly convinced that the function should be assigned to them. First, the members called for a staff paper to review the matter. When the staff recommended that the major responsibility be given to the Department of Health, the matter was referred both to the Council's regular committee on alcoholism and to its citizens advisory committee on alcoholism. After both committees concurred in the staff recommendation, the Council dropped the issue in a typical maneuver for eliminating a source of basic conflict. The Commissioner of Mental Hygiene, who objected to the staff and committee recommendations, suggested that the problem be worked out between the two departments; the Commissioner of

8. Wallace S. Sayre and Herbert Kaufman have pointed out that agencies sometimes "even compete to avoid program assignments that are especially difficult and controversial." See *Governing New York City* (New York, 1960), p. 262.

9. See pp. 30–31.

Health and the others concurred. The struggle essentially was ended by the governor's staff with transfer of the alcoholism program to the Department of Mental Hygiene by the Division of the Budget.

The Council's handling of the question of which department should be responsible for programs for narcotics addicts was too complex to describe here. Suffice it to say that, although it was agreed that the Department of Mental Hygiene should assume responsibility for operation of experimental service facilities for addicts, most of the remaining questions underlying this issue were resolved in the governor's office.

Conflict between Education and Mental Hygiene. For most of a decade there was a difference of opinion between the Education Department and the Department of Mental Hygiene over responsibilities for the vocational rehabilitation of patients in mental hospitals and in schools for the mentally retarded. The Division of Vocational Rehabilitation of the Education Department wanted to expand its services to meet the needs of these patients by placing full-time vocational counselors in mental hygiene facilities. Though some progress was made, there was considerable resistance in the Department of Mental Hygiene to having the Division of Vocational Rehabilitation do so. Although some members of the Council expressed support for closer working relations between the two departments, and occasionally there were reports of the status of negotiations between them, the issue, with one exception, never came before the Council for decision. In this instance, which occurred during the IHRB period, the staff raised the question at a meeting of the Committee on Rehabilitation, and it was suggested that the two agencies strive to improve their relations.

Conflict among Health, Education, and Social Welfare. The 1954 amendments to the federal Social Security Act established a new federal-state program that protected the Old-Age and Survivors' rights of disabled workers through a "disability freeze."[10]

10. Social Security Amendments of 1954, Public Law 761, 83rd Cong., 2d Sess.

The new law set off a round of muted conflict among the Departments of Health, Education, and Social Welfare over which state agency should be designated by the governor to administer the program. The law called for the administering agency to determine the eligibility of injured workers and, thereby, established an important new source of prospective clients for rehabilitation services. The conflict was muted because the Department of Health tried to prevent the program from being assigned to the Division of Vocational Rehabilitation of the State Education Department. The Department of Health felt that if the program were so assigned, there would be great difficulty in persuading the Education Department, and others, of its conviction that the medical expertise of the Department uniquely qualified it to strengthen the medical aspects of the Division's programs.

Although the Department of Health also felt that it was best able to administer the disability freeze, it stood little chance of acquiring this responsibility. Congress had written into the law a preference for state vocational rehabilitation agencies, and federal officials correctly anticipated that most states would agree. Moreover, the second most plausible choice, the Department of Social Welfare, was not much interested. Thus the best course for the Department of Health was to try to discourage the Council from acting, while hoping to persuade the governor of its qualifications for the responsibility or urging that he assign the program to the Department of Social Welfare. However, the issue arose at a time when the Committee on Rehabilitation was reviewing the rehabilitation programs of each agency, and was being urged by the Department of Health to consider the reorganization of state functions. It was hardly the time to ask the Council to drop the issue. Moreover, it was expected that the governor would ask the departments for a recommendation.

In time the Council recommended that the governor designate the Division of the Vocational Rehabilitation as administrator of the new program on a one-year trial basis. Subsequently, however, the Council was notified that this recommendation was unacceptable to the administration because the Division of the

Budget preferred the Department of Social Welfare. The Council then reversed itself and recommended that the responsibility be assigned to that department. The Education Department was not satisfied with this outcome, so that although the issue became dormant it remained a source of potential conflict.

Conflict among Health, Education, Mental Hygiene, and Social Welfare. Development of the state's programs for the mentally retarded caused friction among all four of the core members of the Council. The basic issue, which has national ramifications, and which gained impetus during the Kennedy administration, is whether mental retardation is primarily within the purview of psychiatry and therefore of mental health agencies, or whether it is at least equally the responsibility of other professionals and therefore other agencies. Even though the Department of Mental Hygiene has the greatest responsibility, since it operates the state's custodial and training institutions for severely handicapped, retarded persons, the other three departments also have important functions in this field. The Departments of Health, Education, and Social Welfare particularly have thought that they should play a larger role than the Department of Mental Hygiene has felt they should. Although the issue underlay most Council deliberations on the subject, it emerged directly as an agenda item on only a few occasions, at times with regard to the members' responsibilities for development of a state plan for mental retardation, and at other times in connection with Governor Rockefeller's intention to establish a citizens advisory committee on mental retardation. In each instance the Department of Mental Hygiene did not wish the Council to go into the matter, whereas the other members did. On the first question a direct confrontation of interest was avoided through a strategy of delay, and on the second, the matter was not resolved because agreement could not be reached. (Uncharacteristically, the Council appealed to the Governor's office to settle the latter question.)[11]

11. See pp. 150–52.

Conflict, Cooperation, and the Council's Structure

Given the Council's inclination to avoid conflict, one of the first questions that must be considered is whether the Council could have resolved any of the basic differences among its members, assuming, of course, that a majority of its members wanted it to. The answer clearly is, no. Even if a majority of its members found it desirable to face conflict, the Council could not settle basic differences among its members, for it was powerless. The Council had no legal authority over its members. It even lacked effective, informal inducements or sanctions that could be used coercively, such as the power to provide or withhold funds or highly valuable support for an agency's legislative proposals. Moreover, the Council did not have a constituency to give it support and defend it against attack.[12] Thus, in the absence of direct intervention in its affairs by the governor and possibly by the legislature—which could hardly be counted on and which was rare—the Council was able to deal with conflict only through voluntary agreement of its members.

All that the Council could do was to make recommendations to higher centers of authority. The governor and the legislature could be depended upon to evaluate Council proposals from their own points of view and act accordingly. The individual agencies belonging to the Council also had lines of access to the governor and the legislature that they could utilize with some hope of success to undermine recommendations they deemed unacceptable.

Considering the Council's inclination to eschew conflict and its inability to control its members, a key question becomes unescapable: to what extent did the members cooperate? Certainly the mechanism must have performed a function for its members. The Council existed for two decades, and on the whole was supported by its members remarkably well, if their attendance at meetings is any indication. The commissioners of the four core departments

12. To some extent the Governor's Council on Rehabilitation, a citizens advisory committee established by Governor Rockefeller in 1959, is a constituent group in the area of rehabiiltation. See pp. 158–59.

personally attended almost 80 percent of all meetings of the Council. Also most of the officials familiar with the instrumentality report that they found it the most effective mechanism of its kind in the state government.

The Council agencies cooperated when those having a stake in a matter at hand felt that they would gain more from joint action than they would lose, and when the remaining agencies felt that they would lose nothing of value by assenting. Thus, the members having something at stake cooperated when the things they sought, or wanted to protect, were noncompetitive. Any member agency could hold out without penalty to itself, except possibly that of incurring the displeasure of the other members. The good will or wrath of a sister agency might have influenced a member's conduct, but such sentiments carried little weight when an agency's vital interests were threatened. Members whose interests were unaffected preferred not to interfere with the wishes of the others; also, it cost them nothing to go along, and the favor might be returned. Consequently, the Council shied away from issues involving basic disagreements among its members. To confront charged issues would be to risk that one agency might gain at the expense of another. Since today's winners could be tomorrow's losers, the members had a mutual interest in avoiding such a possibility.

Although the tendency to avoid friction among its members was ingrained in the Council, it did not always prevail. When faced with strong outside pressures, such as from the governor and powerful interest groups, the members sometimes found it necessary to go against the grain. The Council was able to deal with conflict when external pressures made it more costly for the members to avoid a controversial issue than to face it.

However, the pressures upon the members to cooperate were usually light, which meant that the Council seldom had to confront much disagreement.[13] Almost all of the joint decision-making

13. The character of these pressures is a crucial factor that is examined in later chapters. Their influence is considered in an examination of the effect of the agencies' external environment upon the Council and of such

that occurred within the Council was the product of voluntary cooperation, that is, cooperation "based on a sharing of interests," as distinguished from enforced cooperation, or cooperation that "takes place through the overt or implied use of punishments or threats."[14] Even when the cooperative effort was induced by outside pressures, including many instances that involved disagreement among Council members, agreement was voluntary. The external pressures upon the members rarely took the form of demands for cooperative effort within the Council. When joint action was taken, usually the members themselves voluntarily brought the matter to the Council and concluded that such action was desirable. The two most influential outside forces, the governor and the legislature, seldom attempted to determine the choice of agenda items or to influence the course of Council deliberations.

The Council performed some important functions for its members, which helps explain why they cooperated with each other. Through the exchange of information and views, agreement on action by the members, and reports and recommendations to the governor and others, the Council mainly helped the agencies (1) to manipulate their external environment, particularly in mitigating potentially threatening pressures from such sources as the governor, the legislature, and powerful interest groups; (2) to keep an eye on one another, thus reducing the hazards of bureaucratic competition existing outside of the Council; (3) to discover and exploit areas of mutual interest among health programs; and (4) to help each agency head control his own staff.[15]

questions as how the Council can be induced or restructured to handle greater conflict, and how it would respond to increased pressures. See Chaps. 6 and 9.

14. Bertram M. Gross introduces this distinction. Although he applies it to the internal life of organizations, it is equally useful for our purposes. See *The Managing of Organizations* (New York, 1964), I, 267.

15. Although these consequences are distinguishable, they are not achieved by mutually exclusive efforts. For example, in reaching agreement on how to handle an attack upon their programs by an outside interest group, the agencies are likely to learn something about each other's ambitions that may help them avoid fruitless conflict outside the Council.

Control of the Environment

One of the principal functions that the Council performed was to assist its members in manipulating their environment. The benefits that members realized through joint efforts to control their environment seem to have been the most important incentives inducing them to cooperate.[16] For example, 80 percent of the rehabilitation issues that came before the Council during the period studied, and 83 percent of those on which some kind of decision was made, involved attempts to manipulate the external environment (51 of 64, and 39 of 47, respectively).[17] However, only a small proportion of the health matters that concern the agencies in their external relations ever came before the Council. Most of the agencies' dealings with the governor, the legislature, and others are unilateral and are permeated with competition for functions to justify their existence and for resources to sustain organizational life. But when their interests overlapped, and when the benefits to each exceeded the costs, the Council served its members in manipulating their environment in several important ways.

First, the Council enabled the members to take united and thereby more effective action in mitigating threatening pressures and in advancing their interests in the absence of such pressures. For example, they struggled to keep the complaints of interest groups from building up, and they made recommendations to

16. This seems to follow from the fact that the Council members are more dependent upon a common external environment than they are upon each other. For example, although there are important differences among the agencies in the extent to which they are dependent upon a common environment, they are much more dependent upon the governor and the legislature for the legitimation of their purposes and the flow of resources than they are upon each other.

17. An issue is defined as any question implying some kind of decision and therefore is to be distinguished from an exchange of information or views. If brought before the Council, an issue takes the form of an agenda item. However, since an issue may last for several years, it may involve many agenda items. In considering an issue, the members either may take some form of joint action (a decision) or not (no decision). The procedures followed in classifying rehabilitation issues are described in the Appendix.

the governor for the expansion of their programs. By taking joint action, the members also avoided being played against each other. In addition, the Council agencies averted embarrassment to each other in the face of criticism—for example, by avoiding disparate action or conflicting public statements. In some instances, joint decision-making served as a shield against the pressures resulting from decisions that dissatisfied some groups, as in the case of awarding grants to voluntary organizations. By diffusing responsibility, the Council deflected pressures from individual members.

Second, and at least equally important, the Council aided its members in their relations with groups in their environment through extensive exchange of information and views. For example, the members learned from each other the intentions and maneuvers of the governor and of private interest groups, forthcoming legislation, and developments on the national scene. The mechanism served as an informal intelligence center in this respect.

In manipulating the environment, the Council was particularly helpful to its members in warding off and mitigating outside pressures. For instance, 63 percent of the rehabilitation issues that were brought before the Council occasioned attempts to mitigate such pressures (40 of 64). Moreover, 78 percent of all the rehabilitation issues in which efforts were made to control the environment were of this character (40 of 51). In controlling external pressures the members have even voluntarily faced up to some disagreements among themselves. For example, outside influences tipped the scale in favor of joint action on every controversial rehabilitation issue that resulted in a Council decision (4 of 12 such issues). Sometimes, though rarely, agreement was enforced by the potential threat of sanctions, such as when governors referred controversial matters to the Council for resolution. In the field of rehabilitation, this occurred in, at most, 3 percent of all the issues (2 of 64), and 17 percent of the controversial ones (2 of 12). The benefits gained and the problems avoided by the practice of joint response to outside pressures constituted the only effective incentives encouraging Council members to face up to disagreement among themselves.[18]

A few examples of efforts to mitigate outside influences will illustrate. In the first, the advantages of cooperating to control the environment were strong enough to overcome conflicting views among the agencies, albeit with some wavering. Alerted by the staff, Council members in the spring of 1959 rallied in anticipation of repercussions to what they considered unfair criticism of their programs by an eminent university specialist. This authority had criticized, unexpectedly and severely, state services for blind children that were being evaluated in a private study encouraged by interested state agencies. Caught in this dilemma, the members agreed not to issue formal replies, a stand that avoided heating up the controversy and obviated the possibility of any single agency's making damaging or conflicting statements to the press. Each of the interested agencies—Health, Mental Hygiene, Education, and Social Welfare—also agreed to prepare comments on the report's deficiencies and to make recommendations in "anticipation that pressures to implement the recommendations [of the report]" would "be developed during the legislative session."[19] Feeling that the need was "imperative," the chairman said that "such material should be readily available in the event it becomes necessary."[20] The need soon arose, for

18. The environmental pressures that the agencies experience with respect to particular issues, of course, often have substantial implications for their direct relations as well as for their relations with the outside parties from which such pressures emanate. For instance, sharp criticism by a committee of the legislature of the agencies' procedures for referring handicapped persons among their rehabilitation programs affects both the agencies' rehabilitation programs and the agencies' relations with the legislature. Thus, in agreeing on steps to mitigate outside pressures, the members of the Council may have to make changes in the relationships among their programs. Of all the rehabilitation issues that have occasioned responses to outside pressures, 60 percent had substantial implications for the members' direct relations (24 of 40). Moreover, in 56 percent of these issues, the agencies took joint action that involved changes in their direct relations.

19. Minutes of the IHRB, June 2, 1959, p. 1.

20. *Ibid.*, p. 13.

in summer the chairman of a legislative committee officially requested the Council's views on the proposals presented in the report.

Notwithstanding the mounting pressure, Council members had considerable difficulty agreeing on what steps the state should take to improve services to blind children and thus on how to reply to the legislature. All agreed that the services were needed, however. One department was extremely reluctant to assign higher priority to the development of such services, fearing that some of its resources would be diverted thereby from what it considered more important functions. Nevertheless, after about eight months a special subcommitte of the Council reached sufficient agreement so that the Council could reply to the legislature, although the members still could not agree on which department should be responsible for providing the services. The reluctant agency that feared diffusion of its resources, yet the one most favored for the responsibility, finally relented, but only after approximately eight more months of prodding by interested voluntary agencies and groups, and after a special "high level" ad hoc committee of the Council had been formed to resolve the impasse. As a result, agreement was reached on recommendations to the governor, which later were implemented by the establishment of special facilities for emotionally disturbed blind children.

In the foregoing example, the Council enabled the member agencies to take more effective action in dealing with threatening pressures than they could have done individually. It also helped them to avoid being played against one another and needlessly embarrassing each other, as might have happened if they had gone it alone. This episode raises the question of whether the members affected by the issue could have accomplished the same result without the Council. Although these agencies might have cooperated anyway, the Council provided a convenient and accustomed means of taking joint action. In the words of one of the commissioners, the Council "makes it much easier . . . as there is a regular procedure . . . the commissioners do not have to wait until they can get in touch with each other." The Council therefore increased the likelihood both that they would get together and that they would agree. The decisions reached also acquired the formal standing of a body responsible to the governor. Furthermore, the members interested in the issue gained the formal support of the other Council members, an advantage difficult, if not impossible, to come by without the existing mechanism. Finally, had the decisions of the agencies lacked the formal standing of the Council, they would have been more vulnerable to attack as self-serving and defensive.

There are many instances of voluntary efforts by Council members to control external pressures that occasioned little or no conflict among them. In the early 1950's, the Department of Health sought and obtained support for its decision to discontinue certain cerebral palsy research projects that its medical specialists thought were not productive, even though it was under some pressure from a joint legislative commission and interested voluntary agencies to continue them. Recognizing the value of the Council as a shield against the pressures of the special interest groups that objected, the department encouraged the commission to refer the question to the Council for study rather than to appoint a special legislative committee to investigate the need for research in cerebral palsy.[21] The Department of Health also preferred to have the matter considered by a body it could count on to protect its interests, as undoubtedly the Council would, since the other members had little interest in the issue and thus could be expected to agree.

When the Council was reorganized in 1956, it established advisory committees to deal with the problems of chronic alcoholism and mental retardation, partly in response to lively pressures from interested citizen groups. By formally coopting influential representatives of these groups, the Council helped to assuage these pressures at relatively little cost to its members.[22] In the

21. By asking for the Council's advice on the need for the projects in question, the legislature itself was able to deflect some of the pressures it was being subjected to by the same voluntary groups.

22. See p. 31.

words of one of the commissioners, the Council was "a good buffer in protecting the departments against particularly aggressive citizen groups."

During the Harriman administration, Council members found the Council helpful in defending their autonomy against several attempts by the Governor's special assistant on aging to promote establishment, in the executive department of a state commission on aging. They agreed to inform the special assistant of their concern "about the infringement by the [proposed] Commission on responsibilities and actions of various departments, which is not good administrative policy."[23]

At one time the Council even passed a resolution aimed at mitigating federal pressures. The resolution, which the governor welcomed because of a coincidence of interests, was critical of federal agencies for dealing directly with municipalities and thus bypassing state agencies and interfering with supervision of local agencies.

Such examples illustrate voluntary cooperation in the face of outside pressures. On rare occasions, the members have cooperated partly because of the potential threat of sanctions. For example, during the struggle described earlier between the Departments of Health and Social Welfare and the Education Department over which agency should be given the responsibility for administration of the "disability freeze" provisions of the federal Social Security Act, the Council reversed itself when notified that its recommendation was unacceptable to the governor. On another occasion, the Council members recommended that Governor Harriman reorganize the Council and expand its functions by merging it with three independent commissions, even though several of the core members privately and vigorously disagreed.[24] These members acted contrary to their prefer-

23. Minutes of the IHRB, Jan. 29, 1957, p. 7.

24. Memorandum from Dr. Herman E. Hilleboe to Hon. Averell Harriman, on Interdepartmental Council on Human Resources, Feb. 21, 1955. In this memorandum, the Council recommended that the Interdepartmental Health Council be combined with the Mental Health Commission, the Joint Hospital Survey and Planning Commission, and the Youth Commission to form an Interdepartmental Council on Human Relations. See pp. 140–44.

ences in order to accommodate the newly elected Governor when they were informed by the Commissioner of Health that the Governor would welcome such a recommendation. However, in due course the unconvinced members were able unilaterally to persuade the Governor and his staff to limit the scope of the reorganization to include just the Council and one of the three commissions. There are no known cases in which the governor and his staff or the legislature actually imposed sanctions on a member agency or threatened to do so in order to induce cooperative behavior in the Council.

Council members took the initiative to manipulate their environment on many occasions when outside pressures were not present, and thus created and capitalized upon opportunities to extend their influence. For instance, they did so in 17 percent of all the rehabilitation issues that came before the Council (11 of 64) and in 22 percent of these issues that occasioned attempts to manipulate the external environment (11 of 51). However, the agencies found it mutually advantageous to do so only in the absence of basic conflict among themselves, in other words when some or all of the agencies gained and none lost. Such decisions were particularly marked by logrolling. Often they involved the interests of only one or two agencies. Some diverse examples will illustrate the advantages of such cooperation.

Most Council members at one time or another sought and obtained support from the Council for budget requests and for legislative proposals. For example, when in the middle 1950's the Department of Health took measures to convert a declining system of tuberculosis hospitals to timelier, more urgent uses, the Council supported its budget proposals for additional funds to hire rehabilitation personnel. Similarly, at the suggestion of the Commissioner of Insurance, the Council voted in 1963 to endorse several amendments to the State Insurance Law and in 1965 to approve an appropriate resolution in support of a proposed water pollution control program, which the Department of Health and the Rockefeller administration were anxious for the legislature to pass and the voters to implement through an enabling bond issue.

The desire to control the external environment was sometimes clearly articulated. When the Council considered the establishment of a committee on dental health services, for example, the representative of the Department of Correction gave his support, saying that he felt such a committee "might help to convince the Budget" that a dental laboratory it hoped to set up, which had been turned down the previous year, was "a worthwhile project."[25]

On several occasions, Council members tried, usually without success, to draw state budget and civil service officials into meetings at which a case could be made for additional funds or for the upgrading of certain positions. But budget and civil service officials were wary of the agencies' desire to increase their persuasiveness through joint action. On one occasion when Council members were particularly insistent about meeting because of their concern over the large number of unfilled rehabilitation positions in their agencies—vacancies that they attributed to low salaries—budget and civil service representatives conferred before the meeting to plan their strategy and agreed, as one of them reported, "not to be victims of a snow job."

The members also attempted to exert influence over groups other than the governor's staff and the legislature. For example, they cooperated over the years through their committees in sponsoring many educational institutes and conferences throughout the state on mental retardation, alcoholism, etc., that increased their prestige and influence at the grass roots. And they found common cause in influencing some of their sister agencies, as, for example, when they encouraged the state university to increase its output of health manpower, on which they depend, and when they persuaded the State Recreation Council to make special arrangements for the handicapped in state recreational facilities, one of their clienteles.

25. Minutes of the IHRB, Sept. 22, 1959, pp. 9–10.

Relationships Among the Member Agencies

Only a small proportion of the contacts among the member agencies occurred within the Council, namely those that the agencies felt it was to their benefit to initiate. Since the Council was not an instrumentality for the direct management of conflict, such processes as the negotiation and compromise of disagreements were handled outside. Moreover, many routine contacts among the staffs of the agencies also occurred outside the Council, and only some of them stemmed from efforts of the Council.

However, one of the most important functions that the Council performed was to help its members keep an eye on each other and thus make the bureaucratic struggle more predictable and less hazardous. Through such means as the exchange of information and getting reactions to trial balloons, the members increased their understanding of each other's problems, points of view, and intentions. This helped reduce the possibility that the agencies' behavior would be based on misconceptions and that they would needlessly injure one another. A former commissioner of one of the core agencies had in mind the Council's usefulness in this regard when he acknowledged that his department "looked at the Council as a means of clearing lines . . . of avoiding ruptures [with the other members]."

As one would expect, in achieving this benefit, the agencies did not explicitly agree to keep an eye on each other. This function was the subtle product of the need of each agency to learn what it could about another when doing so seemed important to its interests. Likewise, it was the consequence of each member's desire to let the others know something about its own activities and aspirations, usually with the hope of getting approval, or in the hope of eventual reciprocation. And finally, it was a by-product of all of the ways in which the agencies interacted in the Council—for example, of the discussions, studies, reports, and even of the humor and jesting that took place. Consequently, instances of Council behavior that explicitly and dramatically illustrate this indirect management of conflict are somewhat hard to come by.

The exchange of information and views over a wide range of subjects was the principal way in which Council members learned about each other's intentions and likely responses to possible moves on the interdepartmental chess board. Thus, in 1963, when the Commissioner of Mental Hygiene reported on a recent reorganization of his department, a difference of views was revealed between the Departments of Health and Mental Hygiene over the appropriate basis for organization of state regional areas. On another occasion in 1963, the Commissioner of Social Welfare gave his department's position on a commission study of his agency, and informed the Council of the status of implementing legislation. Similarly, in 1959 the Chairman of the Workmen's Compensation Board had informed the Council that a long-awaited report of its operations, requested by the governor, "in no way reflects any of the Board's policies at this time."[26] As part of the process of sharing views, the members frequently discussed their legislative programs, changes in policies, and state and national developments affecting their relationships. They gave something to get something, but did not necessarily reveal all. As one commissioner said, "Each of the members [commissioners] is a gatekeeper . . . he lets out only as much as he feels free and secure to." On one occasion the members were so anxious to find out each other's position on the recommendation of a special study commission, which had called for the transfer of some functions among the agencies, that they agreed to ask the governor's office for permission to exchange the confidential memoranda of their views that had been requested by the governor's office.

The vigor and skill with which the Department of Health fought for its programs, inside the Council and out, enhanced the advantages of cooperation, through which interdepartmental competition becomes more predictable and more containable. The Department of Health thereby increased the usefulness of the Council as a listening post, especially for the other members. On the other hand, it decreased the willingness of the other agencies to cooperate for other purposes. A major thesis of this study

26. Minutes of the IHRB, Jan. 28, 1959, p. 6.

is that the Department of Health's firm resolve in fighting for what it believed in had a great deal to do with stabilizing the Council. As a commissioner reported in confidence, one agency once so feared that the Department of Health would succeed in attaining certain objectives that it called a secret meeting of all commissioners except the Commissioner of Health to warn them about what he felt was a possible "plot." This commissioner apparently supported the continuation of the Council at the time of the Rockefeller reorganization, because he felt "it was better to see what was going on than to be on the outside."

Discovering Areas of Mutual Interest

Another major function of the Council was to help its members discover and exploit areas of mutual interest in the development and administration of their programs—for example, through studies of health needs, the exchange of technical information, and the development of procedures for the referral of patients and clients among their programs. In performing this function, the Council helped its members to make the most of common interests while continuing to compete outside in areas in which their interests conflicted. The members made efforts to work out relationships among their programs in 20 percent of the rehabilitation issues that came before the Council (13 of 64). Consequently, one of the Council's most significant benefits was to help its members maximize cooperation where they had common interests, and minimize conflict by limiting it to the spheres in which their interests truly clashed. In this respect, the Council was an important instrumentality for the indirect management of conflict.

The efforts that were made by the members of the Council to find and exploit areas of mutual interest within their programs is the essence of voluntary cooperation, that is, cooperation not induced by outside pressures and organizational constraints. Such cooperation does not occur when there is basic disagreement among the agencies. For example, the agencies never acted, voluntarily, on a controversial rehabilitation issue mainly involving direct relationships among their programs (3 of 13).

Much of the exchange of information in the Council, particularly the time-consuming studies and continuing discussions conducted within its committees, represented efforts to seek out mutual interests and to arrange mutually advantageous terms of agreement, as well as to feel out the other agencies as a matter of self-interest. A few examples will suffice to illustrate how this relatively undramatic process works.

After overcoming some initial reluctance, the members of the Council found it mutually advantageous to cooperate in the administration of two programs of state aid to facilities serving the handicapped: the Rehabilitation Center Program, and the Sheltered Workshop Support Program. The Council's Committee on Rehabilitation served as a continuing advisory body to the Department of Health and the Education Department in the administration of each of these programs. For example, the Committee participated in the development of criteria for awarding of state funds, the selection of facilities to receive support, and even the approval of key personnel hired to coordinate local rehabilitation programs. In fact, during the last several years of the Council's existence, most of the energies of the Committee on Rehabilitation went into the development of these two programs, and during the years preceding their inauguration much effort was expended in study and discussion of the need for improved and expanded rehabilitation services throughout the state.

There were a number of incentives to cooperate, including Governor Rockefeller's personal interest in rehabilitation and the desire of the members legally responsible for these programs to deflect criticism of their awards of state aid. Apart from these factors, the agencies found a mutual interest in increasing the availability and quality of rehabilitation services for the handicapped. Although interest varied within agencies, each had a clientele that would benefit from greater availability of rehabilitation services. For example, the Division of Vocational Rehabilitation of the Education Department and the local welfare departments had clients who would benefit from referral to facilities specializing in medical rehabilitation, the services of which were fostered by the Department of Health under the Rehabilitation Center Program. Likewise, the patients and clients of the other agencies were aided by the services of the sheltered workshops that were assisted by the Division of Vocational Rehabilitation through its Workshop Support Program.

The discovery of common interests among agencies led to joint training of their professional and management personnel, such as joint participation in a high-level management training program under the auspices of the Civil Service Department. The agencies also found it mutually advantageous to develop better procedures for the referral or transfer of clients and patients. For example, on one occasion the Departments of Health, Social Welfare, and Education worked out arrangements to insure that patients discharged from state tuberculosis hospitals would not be denied public assistance when referred to the Division of Vocational Rehabilitation, an improvement that eliminated an anomaly in eligibility and referral procedures. On another occasion, overlapping interests in improving the quality of educational services to persons confined to state institutions led to agreement on an extensive series of recommendations for improving library services to inmates. Although other factors were influential, the preparation by most of the Council's standing committees of one or more guides to available state services, in such areas as rehabilitation, mental retardation, and emotional disturbance in children, can be attributed in large part to the direct benefits received by the members. By spreading the word about their programs and by learning the dimensions of other's services, they facilitated the exchange of resources, such as clients and information. The values of joint education also helped to inspire the numerous statewide and regional conferences, institutes, and similar meetings that were sponsored by the Council.

Control of Departmental Staffs

The Council was also of value to the heads of the member agencies in controlling their own staffs. Although this function of the Council was much less significant than others, it nevertheless merits comment.

In a sense, agency heads are prisoners of their own staffs, for their lieutenants, who themselves are engaged in maintaining and developing their own units, control the flow of much of the information received at the top echelon. Staff members are in a strategic position to influence how their bosses perceive and respond to issues; moreover, they use this power.

On one occasion, when the commissioners were discussing their departments' legislative proposals, one of them was embarrassed and shocked to learn that another department would vigorously fight "by all the means at its disposal, fair and foul" one of the bills his department was seeking to have introduced in the legislature. Inadvertently or otherwise, this commissioner had not been informed by his staff that another agency would oppose the proposed bill. One of the commissioners said about his colleagues, when he was asked about the value of the Council in controlling their agencies' staffs, that he had the impression that "they sometimes learn things they do not know, and maybe he would some day, too." Since the Council provided the commissioners with an additional source of information, it therefore helped them from being played off against each other by their own lieutenants.

The Disadvantages of the Council

Sometimes the members of the Council felt that it was a potential threat both in their relations with groups in their environment and in their relations with each other.

Participation in the Council opened new channels of interaction with outside agencies, and thus exposed the members to new influences from the environment that could threaten a member agency's autonomy and the security of its functions and resources. For example, an agency sometimes found that its relations with the Council could cause an unfavorable change in the attitudes and expectations of the governor and outside groups toward its activities. Occasionally regular lines of access to the governor or to other influential organizations were weakened or bypassed as a result of Council action. Membership on the Council also created involvements that sometimes could not be shed easily without cost. For example, gaining a reputation for being uncooperative could cause legislators or budget examiners to be less sympathetic to an agency when funds were being provided.

Examples of the disinclination of Council members to work together in manipulating their external environment are more difficult to find than examples of cooperation. This is true partly because it can be costly to be uncooperative. In our society, organizations as well as people are expected to be cooperative, even though cooperation may not serve their best interests. Consequently, Council members, as is true in all organizations, tried to avoid the appearance of being uncooperative even when they were not cooperating. A more important reason, perhaps, is that the external pressures upon the Council, such as those from the governor, were relatively light. As a result, the new channels of interaction opened up by participation in the Council were not very threatening to individual agencies. However, the willingness of the agencies to cooperate in order to control their environment was limited somewhat by the energy with which the Department of Health sought new program responsibilities.

An excellent example of a member's reluctance to be cooperative in attempting to control the external environment is the episode mentioned earlier, in which the Department of Social Welfare was unwilling to have the Council implement Governor Rockefeller's recommendation that it assist in drafting a model code for nursing homes. Believing with some insight that the Department of Health might use the opportunity to present its case for the performance of certain social welfare functions, the Commissioner of Social Welfare demurred. Consequently, Council members agreed to ask for a clarification of the request, which gave the Department of Social Welfare the necessary time to intercede in the Governor's office. In this instance the Department's membership in the Council had led to expectations in the

Governor's office that were threatening to its interests, from which another department hoped to benefit.[27]

On several occasions, some of the members with only peripheral interest in the Council have, in the process of being involved, betrayed a hesitancy to cooperate. The Workmen's Compensation Board's membership in the Council serves as a case in point. In the early 1950's, the governor, in his annual message to the legislature, called upon the Workmen's Compensation Board to arrange for a special study of its rehabilitation program, which had come under heavy fire from both labor and management groups. Partly at the suggestion of the Department of Health, whose advice it had sought in the crisis, the Board successfully encouraged the governor's staff to give the Council a technical advisory role in the development of the study. Yet the Board proceeded to make arrangements with a university to conduct the study without the advice of the Council. This later proved embarrassing to the Board because the study design, as finally reviewed by the other members, was found to be inadequate. Therefore, the Board had to make other arrangements for the conduct of the study. When faced with explaining the Board's reluctance to seek the advice of the Council before a contract was made, the Chairman of the Board said, "there would have been no point in bringing the [Council] . . . into the picture at that stage of the developments."[28]

The Department of Correction was involved in a more muted case of entanglement, which the other members felt it would have preferred to avoid. Originally welcoming the interest of the other members in improving its rehabilitation services to handicapped prisoners, the Department encouraged a Council study of its services and needs. However, this step brought pressures from outside sources, as well as from other Council members, for proposals that threatened top departmental priorities regarding the alloca-

27. This case poses the interesting question of individual members manipulating the Council by influencing outsiders to bring pressures upon the mechanism, which is discussed in Chaps. 5 and 9.

28. Minutes of the IHRB, Feb. 25, 1958, p. 2.

tion of resources. The result was, in the opinion of several of the representatives of the other agencies on the Council, that the Department of Correction felt the Council was interfering in its operations.

The principal costs discouraging cooperation in managing their direct relationships were the potential threats to agencies' functions and resources implicit in joint decision-making. No matter how little autonomy is lost by letting outsiders in on one's affairs, there is always the possibility that vital interests may be compromised. Participating in the Council also exposed an agency to criticism and could reveal some of its weaknesses. It could even cause frictions within an agency—for instance, between the executive and the heads of the agencies' units when Council action was viewed as threatening to its units. In such circumstances, participation in the Council could weaken an executive's control of his agency.

In interpreting the force of such disadvantages, one is reminded of the energetic behavior of the Department of Health, particularly the efforts of the Department, albeit unsuccessful, to have the Council consider the merits of its conviction that the public interest would be better served if it performed some of the medical functions of the other agencies. Since the other members were just as convinced that they should perform these functions, even though in other states the functions may have been assigned to departments of health, they reacted negatively to the attempts by the Department of Health to raise the issues, however obliquely. In general, the discomfort and fears that these efforts left in their wake heightened for the other agencies the disadvantages of cooperating, so that they became less willing to exploit areas of common interest among health programs. Consequently, the extent to which the Council served its members as a vehicle for cooperatively sharing in programs was somewhat retarded.

Examples of the disinclination of the Council members to cooperate in managing their direct interrelationships range from instances of dramatic refusal to unobtrusive unwillingness. The disagreement between the Department of Mental Hygiene and the other agencies over mental retardation planning, described earlier, is a dramatic instance in which a member agency felt strongly that its interests would be threatened by joint decision-making. The Department of Mental Hygiene was anxious to be given the responsibility for development of the state plan for the mentally retarded, but the other agencies, fearful that their interests would not be adequately considered by such an arrangement, opted for the Council. Thus, every time the other members brought up the issue, the Department of Mental Hygiene prevented its being considered through dilatory tactics, while at the same time it strove through regular channels to have the question decided in its favor by the governor. This strategy was successful, even though the Council's Committee on the Mentally Retarded had recommended that the commissioners suggest to the governor that he designate the Council as the state planning agency. Recognizing the Department of Mental Hygiene's adamance, the other members, however unwillingly, acquiesced.

On another occasion, after the reorganization of the Council during the Rockefeller administration, the Department of Mental Hygiene attempted to prevent reestablishment of the committees whose deliberations most affected its interests: mental retardation, emotionally disturbed children, and alcoholism. When the members reexamined the Council's committee structure, the Commissioner of Mental Hygiene suggested "that it might not be necessary to continue all of the committees serving the [Council previously] . . . in view of certain changes in departmental responsibility."[29] This time the Department of Mental Hygiene lost. After a polite delay the committees that it wished abandoned were reorganized. The Department went along with the decision because to have done otherwise would have left the impression that it was uncooperative, since no immediate issue of substance was involved.

Several instances involving the Department of Education illustrate how participation in the Council exposed the members to criticism and led to frictions within an agency. On a number of

29. Minutes of the IHHC, April 26, 1960, p. 3.

occasions, particularly when the Department of Health was attempting to persuade the Council to consider whether or not the medical functions of the Division of Vocational Rehabilitation should be reassigned, weaknesses in the medical phases of the Education Department's vocational rehabilitation program were pointed up. The Department's membership in the Council at times was viewed by several of its units as a potential threat to their autonomy, and at times produced strains between the Commissioner of Education and the heads of some of his units when the commissioner was sympathetic to the views of other Council members. Several officials of the Department of Health reported that such strains sometimes resulted in a breakdown of understanding reached between the Commissioners of Health and Education.

CHAPTER 4

Calculating the Advantages and Disadvantages of Cooperating

IN the previous chapter, in considering how the Council members responded to the advantages and disadvantages of cooperating, no attempt was made to take account of the differences among the agencies. To simplify the exposition, it was also assumed that the agencies act rationally, that is, that they always take appropriate action to further their concept of the public interest, and thus maintain themselves. However, the benefits and costs of cooperating vary from agency to agency, depending upon how perceived interests are affected.

It is now necessary (1) to show how the members' calculations of the assets and liabilities of cooperating with their sister agencies differed and affected their behavior in the Council; (2) to throw light on the rationality of the members' perceptions of participating; and (3) to show how the agencies' unique characteristics as organizations contributed to their views and actions in the mechanism.

The most pronounced dissimilarities existed between the four core members and the other agencies.[1] The core agencies were

1. The "other" agencies considered here were members between 1953 and 1960: the Department of Labor; the Workmen's Compensation Board; the Department of Correction; and the Division of Parole; after 1960 they were represented on some of the committees of the Council. Also included

much more interested in the Council than the other agencies, principally because of the greater magnitude and interrelatedness of their health functions. They stood to gain or lose much more from involvement.

There was also significant variation among the core members in their estimation of the values of Council participation. These differences, however, appear to have been related less to differences in the range and the interdependence of the members' health functions than to a complex of organizational characteristics that influenced their perceptions of the values of cooperating. Factors like changes in agency functions, organizational structure, and agency outlook affected their judgments. Thus, the Department of Health, an influential agency that energetically sought new programs largely because of the changing character of public health functions, tended to be sanguine about the value of the Council. By contrast, the Departments of Mental Hygiene and Social Welfare were inclined to weigh heavily the costs of involvement, owing to their unique characteristics. For example, most of the energies of the Department of Mental Hygiene went into the operation of geographically isolated and highly autonomous institutions for the mentally ill. The result was an insularity of outlook that precluded much intercourse with other agencies. Similarly, as a relatively disunited agency caught in a crossfire of political pressures, the Department of Social Welfare was easily threatened by the risks of participating in the Council. And the last of the foursome, the State Education Department, viewed the Council equivocally. Possessing many of the characteristics

are the Insurance Department, which became a member in 1960. Although the Joint Hospital Survey and Planning Commission and the Youth Commission also were members for part of the period between 1953 and 1960, they are excluded from the analysis because the Hospital Commission had a unique status, as its executive director served as secretary to the Council during the IHC phase, and because the Youth Commission was a member for about one year. Moreover, neither was an operating agency in the usual sense. The commissioners of most of the four core agencies served on both Commissions. See pp. 27–33 for the historical background of the Council's membership.

of a university detached from the world, the Department tended to speak with conflicting voices in calculating the assets and liabilities of cooperating.

The members were also sensitive to each other's behavior. Here the Department of Health had the dominant effect, for its behavior profoundly enhanced some of the factors that contributed to the members' calculations and behavior. In particular, the energy and determination with which the Department pursued its goals heightened the inherent cautiousness and fears of the other members, at one time to such a degree that two of the agencies would have liked to see the Council disbanded if this could have been accomplished without injury and embarrassment to themselves.[2]

However, the views of the agencies gradually altered over the years, as some of their characteristics changed, and particularly because the restlessness of the Department of Health waned. Paradoxically, the agencies were probably more in accord in their attitudes toward the Council during its final days than at any other time during the life of the mechanism. The advantages and disadvantages of participating in the Council rested in fairly close balance, and ambivalence was the hallmark of the agencies' attitudes at the end. Although this ambivalence was most marked then, it was always present.

The strength of the core agencies' interest was expressed in various ways, but it was most graphically reflected in their greater attendance at meetings, and in their general dominance of the Council. Furthermore, the primacy of the core members was accepted by the other agencies without serious question.[3]

When one compares the attendance of the core members with that of the other agencies the results are striking. As shown in Table 1, the core members as a group attended 96 percent of all the Council meetings over the life of the Council, whereas the other agencies, as a group, participated in 77 percent of the meet-

2. See p. 148.
3. The governor's office also has taken a similar view. See Chap. 6.

ings held during the period they were members. Furthermore, each of the core agencies was represented more often at meetings than the other agencies, with the exception of the Education Department, which was surpassed only by the Department of Insurance. For example, the core agencies' attendance ranged from 100 percent of all Council meetings, in the case of the Department of Health, to 94 percent, in the case of the Education Department. By comparison, the proportion of Council meetings participated in by the other agencies, excluding the Department of Insurance, ranged from 80 percent, in the instance of the Department of Labor, to 64 percent, in the instance of the Division of Parole. The Department of Insurance was represented at 98 percent of all the Council meetings from the time it became a member in 1960.

The disparity in the participation of the two groups of agencies in the Council becomes even more evident in terms of the attendance of the agency heads at meetings. As Table 2 shows, the heads of the core members, taken as a group, attended almost 80 percent of all the meetings, a truly astonishing record.[4] By contrast, the chief executives of the other agencies participated in fewer than 20 percent of the meetings. Furthermore, there are no exceptions to this sharp divergence between the groups. The core member whose head attended the fewest meetings, the Education Department, was represented by its commissioner almost 70 percent of the time. By contrast, the highest performer among the other agencies, the Workmen's Compensation Board, was represented by its chairman at only 24 percent of the meetings. These patterns of agency participation in Council meetings prevailed during all phases of the Council's existence, as Tables 1 and 2 show. Furthermore, they were reflected in the meetings of the committees of the Council, although to a less marked

4. One of the core commissioners confided to the author that Governor Harriman's secretary was amazed that the commissioners personally attended Council meetings and felt that it was a waste of their time. This commissioner also acknowledged that he "didn't go to other interdepartmental meetings and boards, of which there are many."

degree. To illustrate: each of the core members, with few exceptions, ranked ahead of all of the other agencies in attending the meetings of each committee, except for the regional committees (rehabilitation).[5]

The four core departments also had the main voice in the Council since its inception, even during the period between 1953 and

TABLE 1

PERCENTAGE OF COUNCIL MEETINGS ATTENDED BY EACH COUNCIL AGENCY, DURING THE THREE PHASES OF THE COUNCIL[a]

1946–1964

	Council Phase			
Agency	All Three	IHC	IHRB	IHHC
(Number of Meetings)	(148)	(68)	(39)	(41)
All Core Agencies	*96%*	*95%*	*98%*	*100%*
Health	100%	100%	100%	100%
Social Welfare	99	99	97	100
Mental Hygiene	97	96	95	100
Education	94	87	100	100
(Number of Meetings)	(64)	(25)	(39)	–
All Other Agencies[b]	*73%*[c]	*69%*	*76%*	–
Labor	80%	71%	87%	–
Workmen's Compensation	80	79	82	–
Correction	70	58	80	–
Parole	64	79	56	–
(Number of Meetings)	–	–	–	(41)
Insurance	–	–	–	98%

[a] Based on Council minutes covering the period December, 1946, to December, 1964. Minutes of all but two or three meetings were extant.

[b] These agencies were members of the Council from September, 1953, to March, 1960, except for the Insurance Department, which has been a member since March, 1960. Excluded are the Joint Hospital Survey and Planning Commission and the Youth Commission. See Note 1, p. 75.

[c] With the Insurance Department included becomes 77 percent.

5. The regional committees (rehabilitation) are discussed in Chap. 7.

TABLE 2

PERCENTAGE OF COUNCIL MEETINGS ATTENDED BY THE EXECUTIVE HEADS OF EACH COUNCIL AGENCY, DURING THE THREE PHASES OF THE COUNCIL[a] 1946–1964

Agency	Council Phase			
	All Three	IHC	IHRB	IHHC
(Number of Meetings)	(148)	(68)	(39)	(41)
All Core Agencies	*78%*	*75%*	*83%*	*77%*
Health	85%	82%	95%	83%
Social Welfare	80	79	87	73
Mental Hygiene	79	78	74	85
Education	69	63	74	66
(Number of Meetings)	(64)	(25)	(39)	–
All Other Agencies[b]	*17%*[c]	*27%*	*11%*	–
Workmen's Compensation	24%	34%	18%	–
Parole	17	28	10	–
Labor	14	24	8	–
Correction	14	24	8	–
(Number of Meetings)	–	–	–	(41)
Insurance	–	–	–	22%

[a] Based on Council minutes covering the period December, 1946, to December, 1964. Minutes of all but two or three meetings were extant.

[b] These agencies were members of the Council from September, 1953, to March, 1960, except for the Insurance Department, which has been a member since March, 1960. Excluded are the Joint Hospital Survey and Planning Commission and the Youth Commission. See Note 1, p. 75.

[c] With the Insurance Department included becomes 18 percent.

1960, when the Council's membership reached a high of 10 members. Their prominence continued from the reorganization in 1960, when all of the agencies except the core members were dropped and the Department of Insurance was added, until the Council was disbanded in 1967.

The core agencies dominated the Council in many ways. First, they initiated most of the Council's action and business. The core agencies initiated 78 percent of the rehabilitation issues that were brought before the Council by a member (28 of 36), the remaining 22 percent having been initiated by the other agencies (8 of 36).[6] Second, the core members were interested in many more of the areas of concern that had been considered by the Council. For instance, each of the core agencies ranked ahead of the other members in the number of rehabilitation issues that involved their interests. Third, they always held the reins of the Council. Thus, starting with the IHRB phase, 1956–1960, when the Council was required to elect its chairman, the position was rotated annually among the core members. Prior to this time, the Commissioner of Health had been the chairman, ex officio. Although the 1960 reorganization precluded the possibility of passing the chairmanship on to one of the other agencies, it is extremely doubtful that any of the others would have welcomed the responsibility. In fact, the chairmanship entered a second round of rotation among the core agencies when the Department of Insurance became a member, although the executive order under which the Council then operated made that department just as eligible to lead the Council as any other member. Fourth, the core members were also represented on more of the Council's committees than any of the other agencies. A further indication of what, in effect, was two classes of membership was the failure of the commissioners of the core agencies to invite the heads of the other agencies to join them at informal luncheons, for many years held immediately following the meetings of the Council. An exception was made in the case of the Superintendent of Insurance after the reorganization in 1960, but the Superintendent usually

6. The core members also had many more opportunities to bring up rehabilitation issues since the Council was actively interested in the subject after 1953; the noncore agencies' participation in this program was limited mainly to representation on the Committee on Rehabilitation, except during the four-year period when most of them also were members of the Council, 1956–1960. (See pp. 27–33 for changes in the membership.) However, the core agencies also initiated 79 percent of the rehabilitation issues brought up by members that first were raised in the Committee on Rehabilitation. These computations exclude issues initiated by the Council staff.

TABLE 3

ESTIMATED OPERATING EXPENDITURES OF SELECTED COUNCIL MEMBERS FOR HEALTH PURPOSES AS A PERCENTAGE OF THEIR TOTAL OPERATING EXPENDITURES DURING 1964–1965[a]

Agency	Amount of Expenditures: For Health	Amount of Expenditures: Total	Health Expenditures as a Percentage of Total Expenditures
Mental Hygiene	$298,920,000	$ 298,920,000	100.0%
Social Welfare	108,573,000[b]	588,890,000	18.4
Health	105,765,000[c]	105,765,000	100.0
Education	12,678,960[d]	1,196,100,000	1.1
Insurance	600,000[e]	7,612,000	7.9
Labor	4,691,797[f, g]	94,343,573	5.0
Workmen's Compensation	3,655,192[h]	11,790,941	31.0
Correction	2,750,000[i]	54,798,521	5.0
Parole	200,000[j]	5,636,418	3.5

[a] Represents expenditures from all sources of funds, including those for local assistance payments to units of local government, but excludes state expenditures for capital construction. Method of computation recommended by the Division of the Budget, Executive Department, with the assistance of some of the agencies, but the definition of health purposes is the author's. The period is April 1, 1964, to March 31, 1965.

[b] Includes all of the separately identified amounts for health purposes, of which the bulk is medical assistance to the aged, disability determinations under federal Social Security provisions, and the operating expenses of the Division of Medical Services; therefore somewhat underestimates the total expenditures for health purposes.

[c] Supervision of funeral directing, which it is estimated is under $500,000, might have been excluded.

[d] Includes vocational rehabilitation, pupil personnel services, and an estimated amount for health professional regulation. Excludes unidentifiable amount for scholarships, fellowships, and scholar incentive awards paid to students in the health professions.

[e] Includes supervision and rate regulation of health insurance.

[f] Includes industrial safety services, industrial hygiene, the Board of Standards, and an estimated amount for special placement of the handicapped.

[g] Excludes Workmen's Compensation Board, which is a part of the Department.

did not attend.[7] In conclusion, there is no evidence that the dominance of the Council by core members was ever seriously challenged, let alone questioned, by any of the other agencies. On the contrary, it seems to have been accepted by them as a proper reflection of the core agencies' greater stakes in the Council.

Two factors seem to have contributed most to the deeper interest of the core members in the Council: the greater magnitude and the greater interrelatedness of their health functions. The size and relative magnitude of the health programs of the Council agencies varied widely, but the most striking differences occurred between the programs of the core members and those of the other agencies. To illustrate: all of the activities of the Departments of Mental Hygiene and Health have a health focus, whereas only a segment of the programs of the other agencies do. As shown in Table 3, the total expenditures of the agencies for health purposes in 1964–1965 ranged from approximately $299 million, spent by the Department of Mental Hygiene, to about $200 thousand, spent by the Division of Parole. Similarly, the share of the agencies' budgets devoted to health activities varied during the same period from a high of 100 percent, in the case of the Departments of Mental Hygiene and Health, to a low of about 1 percent, in the instance of the Education Department. Yet, notwithstanding this variation, each of the core members spent more money for health purposes than each of the other agencies. Furthermore, with the exception of the State Educa-

[h] Represents 31 percent of the total expenditures of the Board, which is the proportion of total payments to claimants by employers and insurance companies for medical and rehabilitation purposes ($55,045,000 of $177,-689,000). This probably overestimates the Board's expenditures for health.

[i] Includes expenditures for medical purposes to which an estimated amount (ca. 25 percent) has been added for supportive services and indirect expenditures.

[j] Includes program for mental defectives, specialized narcotics program, mental health unit, and estimated amount of indirect expenditures.

7. The fact that the meetings of the Council are held in Albany and the office of the Superintendent of Insurance is located in New York City has discouraged the Superintendent from accepting the invitation of his colleagues, particularly since he rarely attends the meetings himself.

tion Department's budget of well over $1 billion, most of which is appropriated for State aid to local school districts, the core agencies also tended to contribute a larger share of their total resources to health programs than did the other agencies.

Major differences also existed among the agencies in the interdependence of their health functions, that is, in the extent to which the programs and policies of one agency had ramifications in another. However, the health responsibilities of the four core members, especially the Departments of Health, Mental Hygiene, and Social Welfare, were much more intimately linked than those of the other agencies. A look at the committee structure of the Council shows that they had more areas of interdependence. The core agencies had strong ties in the areas of rehabilitation, nursing, mental retardation, aging, alcoholism, and narcotics addiction. These subject areas were the focus of interest of the most active and long-standing committees. By contrast, the other agencies had fewer points of interdependence, as reflected in the fact that they participated in fewer committees than the core agencies. To illustrate: the Department of Correction's interest in health is confined to its responsibilities for the inmates of state prisons, including prisons for the criminally insane, which brings the Department in close contact with the Department of Mental Hygiene. The Department of Correction's interest in health, therefore, has been limited largely to maintenance of a unique incarcerated population, although it has extended its concerns to narcotics addiction, alcoholism, mental retardation, and rehabilitation. The interest of the Division of Parole in health is also confined to the same population group, but is even more limited in scope, since the Division does not have responsibility for domiciling an inmate population. The Division is concerned principally with the health of parolees because of the effect that their health may have upon their capacity to make a satisfactory adjustment within society. Consequently, the Division is particularly interested in rehabilitation. The Department of Labor has responsibilities for regulating conditions of private employment to protect the health and safety of workers, and its Employment

Service helps the severely disabled to find jobs. The Department, therefore, is particularly concerned with industrial medicine, which brings it into contact with the Department of Health, and with rehabilitation of the disabled. The health interests of the Workmen's Compensation Board derive from the latters' adjudication of the claims of workers upon employers for medical services and compensation for injuries related to their employment. Although this involves the agency in medical affairs, the Board provides no direct services to clients other than to protect the rights of injured workers. In recent years, it has required employers and their agents, the insurance companies underwriting workmen's compensation policies, to pay for rehabilitation services whenever the prognosis is favorable. The Board's interest in the Council, therefore, was largely limited to rehabilitation.

There were also relationships among the agencies' health responsibilities that were not considered in the Council, as will be shown, but these too were more extensive in the case of the core agencies than the others.[8]

In conclusion, the four core agencies played a much larger role in the Council than the other agencies, for they stood to gain or lose the most from doing so. They showed the strongest interest, as a result of the absolute and relatively greater magnitude of their health functions and the greater interdependence of their responsibilities. However, the behavior of the other agencies cannot be accounted for entirely by these differences. Other factors such as agency outlook, organizational structure, and power were influential. For instance, because the core agencies were much larger and more powerful, the other members seem to have been somewhat reluctant to get too involved with them. A former state official who attended Council meetings during this period called them "the power commissioners." Also, the efforts of the Department of Health to get the Council to resolve agency differences was at its height during the time that most of the other agencies were members. Because these agencies played a second-

8. See Chap. 8 and pp. 36–39.

ary part in the Council, this discussion has been limited to consideration of the most important factors that contributed to their outlook and behavior. For the same reason, no attempt will be made to compare the differences in the outlook of these agencies or to consider the rationality of their actions. It seems that they not only found membership in the Council of little value, but, because of what they regarded as potential risks to their autonomy, probably a net disadvantage as well. Like some of the core agencies, they, too, seem to have feared for their interests.

Before showing how the core members individually calculated the advantages and disadvantages of cooperating, it is necessary to be more explicit about the concept of rationality employed in this study. Implicit in the analysis of the agencies' response to the possibilities of cooperating, presented in Chapter 3, is the assumption that agency representatives necessarily expressed a view of the public interest that took account of their agencies' maintenance and enhancement needs, and, further, that they strove to take appropriate action to advance or defend these interests. In other words, they acted rationally to sustain their organizations. Certainly, the findings presented earlier strongly suggest that the commissioners acted with considerable rationality in these terms.[9]

This conception of rationality does not exclude nondeliberative action. Much of the behavior of the commissioners probably was intuitive rather than calculating. It was nonetheless rational with respect to the objective of organizational survival, however latent that goal might have been in consciousness.

Yet since organizations are composed of people, they do not act with perfect rationality owing to the limitations of human cognition and judgment, which, of course, are universal.[10] Fur-

9. In their monumental study of New York City, Wallace S. Sayre and Herbert Kaufman found that "agency heads usually become adept at calculating the gains and costs of various courses of action." See *Governing New York City* (New York, 1960), p. 263.

10. Consideration of theories of cognition and decision-making are outside the scope of this study. The reader is referred to James G. March and Herbert A. Simon, *Organizations* (New York, 1958) and to David Braybrooke and Charles E. Lindblom, *A Strategy of Decision* (New York, 1963).

thermore, the commissioners and their staffs are susceptible to a variety of influences, peculiar to their agencies, that affect their perceptions of their agencies' interests and ultimately their decisions, some of which are functional and some dysfunctional for maintenance of their agencies.[11] For example, such organizational factors as the degree of autonomy of an agency's constituent units and its professional orientation not only may contribute to its cohesiveness but also may diminish its capacity to adapt successfully to a changing environment. Thus, the historic isolation of the state institutions for the mentally ill has promoted an insularity of viewpoint in the Department of Mental Hygiene that, as will be shown, led commissioners and their staffs to be unnecessarily wary of cooperating in the Council. As James March and Herbert Simon have pointed out, "The organizational and social environment in which the decision maker finds himself determines what consequences he will anticipate, what ones he will not; what alternatives he will consider, what ones he will ignore."[12] These factors make themselves felt upon the perceptions and decisions of organization members in what March and Simon call their "definition of the situation."[13]

There were substantial differences in the four core members' calculations of the benefits and costs of participating in the Council. During most of the life of the Council, the Department of Health looked very favorably upon the advantages of membership, whereas the other three departments were much less sanguine. This outcome is attributable to a complex of factors, including the nature of the agencies' health responsibilities, organizational structure, power, outlook, and reputation, which together made the needs of each unique in some respects, and which colored the perceptions and behavior of the agencies' leaders.

11. Robert K. Merton points out the importance of recognizing the dysfunctional as well as functional consequences of social structures. See *Social Theory and Social Structure* (rev. ed., New York, 1957), pp. 19–85.

12. March and Simon, p. 139.

13. *Ibid.*

The Department of Health

The Department of Health had the greatest impact upon the Council. Although it was the smallest of the four core members, measured by budget size, its future-mindedness, its vigorous behavior, and its strong influence with governors and others profoundly affected the way the other members viewed the assets and liabilities of Council participation.

Of all the members, the Department of Health had the most positive and favorable attitude toward the Council, although this view changed in later years.[14] Commissioners of Health and their immediate staffs looked upon the Council as a mechanism by which they, at least in part, could persuade others of their conviction that the health needs of people in our time require that public health agencies play a much larger and more dynamic role. In particular, they hoped to make headway in getting other agencies to accept the view that the Department of Health was best qualified to assume certain of the health responsibilities assigned to other Council members. Almost always on the offensive and usually confident that it eventually would triumph, the Department seldom, if ever, feared that its interests would suffer as a result of Council involvement. On the contrary, coordination, as represented by the Council, was considered good politics in the broadest sense of the term, for the leaders of the Department welcomed the Council as an additional means of pursuing their objectives. A member of the governor's staff was of the opinion that the Department thought highly of the Council because it offered "an alternative to a frontal assault, with its hazards of stepping on the toes of the other departments." Moreover, according to its leaders, the Department not only hoped that it could realize some of its objectives through cooperative action, but it also believed that its disagreements with the other agencies made

14. This chapter is concerned mainly with the behavior of the departments over the long span of the Council and less with the implications of the changes that have occurred in their outlook, particularly those in recent years.

it all the more important to keep open the lines of communication in order to avoid needless antagonism.[15]

Consequently, the Department of Health had a relatively conscious strategy in approaching the Council, which was to bring up as many issues as it could in the expectation that at least some of them would be resolved according to Department objectives. As a member of the Department put it in earthier language, "Every once in awhile we would put out some bait and catch a fish." Thus, for example, the Department directly initiated 56 percent of the rehabilitation issues that were brought up by the members (20 of 36), the remaining 44 percent having been raised by the other agencies (16 of 36).[16] As part of this strategy, the Department repeatedly encouraged and pressed the Council to see these issues through to a conclusion. In fact, the Department pushed the Council about as much as a member could, though seldom beyond the informal rules of the game, as will be shown later.[17]

Throughout much of the life of the Council, the Department of Health expected to derive more from the mechanism than it did. Thinking that it could make important gains, such as Council support for the transfer to its purview of medical functions assigned to the Departments of Education and Social Welfare, the Department met with disappointment. In looking back over the years, a current leader of the Department acknowledged that he "rather doubted the Department has gained anything with respect to taking over functions." In effect, the agency misjudged the Council's capacity to deal with controversial matters. Partly as a result, there has been a decline in recent years of the Department's optimism regarding the usefulness of the Council. The

15. Reformulating Georg Simmel's propositions, Lewis A. Coser argues that "conflict acts as a stimulus for establishing new rules, norms, and institutions, thus serving as an agent of socialization for both contending parties." See *The Functions of Social Conflict* (New York, 1956), p. 128.

16. The procedures followed in classifying rehabilitation issues are described in the Appendix.

17. See Chap. 5.

Department's functions also have been expanded substantially in recent years though not through help from the Council.

The Department's strategy of pressing the Council to deal with controversial matters also was somewhat dysfunctional for its purposes. Rather than contributing to cooperation among the members of the Council in areas in which they had common interests, this strategy tended to have the opposite effect, since the other agencies were much less vigorous in pursuing their interests. Recognizing the objectives of the Department of Health, the other members assumed the defensive, which made them wary and hesitant to enter into agreements for fear their interests would suffer. As a representative of the Department of Health indicated, the other commissioners frequently attended the meetings themselves, "to be sure they didn't lose any fingers. . . . They didn't send underlings to bargain away part of their empires." Thus, the net effect of the Department's behavior was to dampen the interest of the other agencies in the Council, which, as later chapters will show, was reflected in the business that they brought to the Council and in the support that they gave it in moments of crisis.

The Department's strategy may however be considered successful in the larger sense that it was part of a broader and continuing effort to develop support for acquiring functions that it believed itself best qualified to perform. Although its hopes in the Council were not fulfilled, the Department found that the Council was one of several means by which it could increase pressure for the realignment of certain health functions. Thus the Department's strategy contributed to the growth of its responsibilities however dysfunctional this strategy may have been for the Department's objectives within the mechanism.

Several factors contributed to the Department of Health's forceful behavior and to its overestimation of what it could expect to derive from Council membership. Although the smallest of the core agencies, the Department was one of the most powerful members, in terms of its ability to influence governors, legislators, and private interest groups. As perhaps the most cohesive agency, held together by a corps of highly trained and respected public health physicians who are accustomed to strong leadership, the Department enjoyed an outstanding reputation for effectiveness in all quarters. As the state's generalist agency in health, the Department has been unusually responsive to changing needs for governmental health programs. It has been quick to seize and create opportunities to modify and expand existing programs and take on new responsibilities. The Department also was the first to embrace the program planning and management techniques that came into favor shortly after World War II. Even its adversaries speak very highly of its abilities and long-range views. Moreover, unlike other Council agencies run by highly trained professionals, the Department of Health has energetically presented its case to those who could potentially be of assistance. Thus it has frankly courted the centers of power and willingly cultivated constituencies.

Much of the impetus for the energy and effectiveness of the Department of Health is related to the changing character of public health programs. Since the beginning of this century, and particularly since World War II, the control of communicable diseases, the traditional raison d'être for public health agencies, has largely been accomplished. In its place a whole range of newer problems, such as chronic illness, air and water pollution, and the quality and general availability of medical services, have intensified. However, the Department has not had clear title to many of the newer functions, for some either have been claimed by other agencies, or for historical reasons have fallen in other jurisdictions. A student of the Department said of public health, "the scope and boundaries of no public function are more in dispute, both as to what the responsibilities of government should be and how these responsibilities should be divided and executed."[18] Recognizing the exigencies of survival, the Department

18. Morris Schaefer, "Area and Function in the Administration of Public Health in New York State," unpublished doctoral dissertation, Syracuse University, 1962, p. 22. Schaefer also said of the Department of Health: "It has absorbed such broad changes in function as the decline of tuberculosis and communicable diseases and the rise in the importance of chronic diseases and new environmental health problems. It is justifiably regarded as the leading agency in its field in the United States" (p. 372).

of Health over the last several decades has been engaged in the task of rebuilding itself as a vital and secure agency of state government by pulling together and developing various changing health functions. A Department official put the problem this way, "We decided we were not going to get much business being an epidemiological fire department, waiting around to put out epidemics." Since some health-related functions were assigned to other agencies and the claim to still other functions was in dispute, the circumstances demanded a policy of expansion, which necessarily has increased the competition among the state agencies with health responsibilities. The underlying basis for this competition was well recognized by the other departments. As an influential agency in "need of new fields to conquer," to use the words of a former Department of Health official, the agency has taken a long view of the public interest and pursued it vigorously.

As a relatively well-knit agency, the Department of Health also has enjoyed some advantages in exercising influence that have encouraged it to be energetic. Because of their authority, Commissioners of Health had greater freedom to maneuver in the Council than the heads of the other agencies. They were better able to speak for and commit their agency, and even to reverse themselves, when it was in the interests of the Department to do so. Moreover, the staff of the Department had the security and assurance of positive objectives in their dealings with their counterparts on Council committees. The Department also benefited from direct and clear lines of responsibility to the governor, which it exploited in its relations with the other members. The Commissioner of Health is appointed by the incoming governor, with the consent of the state senate, for the length of the gubernatorial term. Unlike the Commissioners of Social Welfare and Education, the Commissioner of Health does not have to contend with a supervisory board in his relations with the governor and legislature. The sometimes dramatic and frequently greater political appeal of public health programs, compared with programs for the mentally ill and the indigent, also weighs heavily in its favor. Although the popularity of governmental programs changes (as seen in the increased interest in mental illness and mental retardation, and most recently in poverty), the Department of Health has benefited from social and political changes that it has exploited to its advantage.

Another agency strength, an unusually able professional staff, seems to have contributed to the Department's behavior, and, as acknowledged by its own spokesmen, to its overestimation of what it could expect to gain from participation in the Council. The personnel of the Department of Health gave the impression, particularly at the committee level of the Council, that only physicians can speak with authority on health matters. Sometimes the Department's staff also gave the other agencies the feeling that they believed the Department possessed most of the medical expertise in state government. This tended to annoy some of the other members, with the result that they were less willing to cooperate. In commenting on the Department of Health's behavior in the early days of the Committee on Rehabilitation, when the Department was subjecting the Council to considerable pressure, a representative of another agency said, "They [the representatives of the Department of Health] also forgot the other agencies had MDs." As interviews show, many of the representatives of the other Council members felt that the Department of Health staff had too high an opinion of itself; nevertheless these representatives acknowledged a high regard for the competence of the Department. Without question, differences in outlook and status deriving from the varied professional backgrounds of their staffs affected the behavior of the agencies and their reaction to each other in the Council.

The Department of Mental Hygiene

The attitude of the Department of Mental Hygiene toward the Council was mainly negative; its representatives tended to dwell upon the disadvantages of cooperating. A top official of the Department commented on the outlook of a former commissioner as follows: "He betrayed his lack of enchantment about its worthwhileness to our Department . . . he just went through the motions." This point of view, however, changed as the Department moved away from its past insularity in response to the trend toward treating the mentally ill in their home communities where possible, rather than in isolated institutions.[19] In the words of a representative of another agency, "The Department has come a long way from its insularity."

Although it is the third largest agency in the state, measured by budget size, and is by far the largest employer and largest health agency, the Department of Mental Hygiene generally regarded the Council as a potential threat to its interests. Along with the Department of Social Welfare, it was especially sensitive to the forcefulness of the Department of Health. A member of the governor's office said that in his judgment of all the departments, the Department of Mental Hygiene was "most jealous of its functions . . . and had the greatest bureaucratic paranoia." However, the Department's reaction to the Department of Health was more nearly that of a slumbering Goliath irritated by a pesky boy than that of a man beset with fear. Although the Department's posture toward the Council was negative, it was the negativism of a strong agency seeking to avoid entangling relationships. Consequently, the strategy of the Department in the Council was largely one of disengagement. This was most evident in the first few years after the reorganization of the Council in 1960 in the Rockefeller administration; as, for instance, in the unsuccessful efforts of the Commissioner of Mental Hygiene to prevent the Council from reestablishing the committees most concerned with his agency's programs.

Throughout most of the years of the Council, the Department of Mental Hygiene tended to feel that its interests were endan-

19. The state plans for service to the mentally retarded and to the mentally ill developed recently under the aegis of the Department recommended that the role of the Council be expanded and strengthened in both of these areas. See *A Plan for a Comprehensive Mental Health and Mental Retardation Program for New York State, Vol. I, Report of the Mental Health and Mental Retardation Sections of the State Planning Committee* (Albany, N. Y., July 1, 1965), pp. 21, 53, 108, 110.

gered by participation. In focusing upon the disadvantages, the Department was inclined to overlook potential benefits. But there certainly is no evidence that the agency ever lost anything of value. It was, for example, victorious in retaining under its aegis all of the programs sought by the Department of Health, and the Department succeeded in preventing the other members from gaining control through the Council of planning in the area of mental retardation. The Council's inability to handle controversial issues meant that no department's interests were ever seriously jeopardized. Therefore it seems that the Department's strategy of trying to disengage was unnecessary. Furthermore, insofar as disengagement was attempted, it was not very effective. For one, it was not a team effort, as was the strategy of the Department of Health. For another, it tended to be a rearguard, foot-dragging effort, reflective of an underlying reluctance rather than of positive conviction.

Because of the agency's enormous size, one cannot attribute the largely negative and defensive attitude of the Department of Mental Hygiene toward the Council to a lack of power. Although its reputation suffered at times during the Council's life span, especially during the latter years of the Dewey administration, the Department has always enjoyed considerable influence. Furthermore, for years it has been one of the most outstanding mental health agencies in the country. It was a leader in the introduction over a decade ago of revolutionary techniques of drug therapy. However, its power often has taken the form of inertia.

The general outlook and behavior of the Department in large measure has reflected the way in which New York, as well as other states, traditionally has coped with the mentally ill. The long-standing practice of incarcerating people with mental illness in huge geographically isolated state institutions has produced an insular attitude that pervades the department. A representative of another agency described the personnel of the agency as "having their own big cocoon." Unfavorable public attitudes toward mental illness and psychiatrists, largely reflecting ignorance and fear, have contributed to this insularity, for society has preferred to avoid the problems of the emotionally disturbed. Rarely in the past has the public shown much interest in the problem of the mentally ill, except when a scandal, usually traceable in part to inadequate public support, broke out. Furthermore, until the last decade, the psychiatrists who have run the Department of Mental Hygiene have been unable to show much for their labors. The overwhelming proportion of those committed to state hospitals have stayed for life. This result hardly has been conducive to public confidence or to esteem in professional circles. Thus, until the advent of tranquilizers and other drugs, most of the external and internal forces playing upon the Department tended to cut it off from the mainstream of bureaucratic life.

In part the professional cement that holds the Department together—the medical specialty of psychiatry—has contributed to the Department's lack of experience and temperament for outside relations. As perhaps the most esoteric medical specialty, psychiatry is a much narrower field than public health. The psychiatrist administrator, until recently, has been cut off from the field of medicine and has lacked formal education in administration and community relations and has therefore lacked an understanding of the relationship between administration and the political process. Therefore, more than most professionally trained people, he has been inclined to regard involvement in the political realm as unprofessional and accordingly to be avoided.

The internal structure of the Department of Mental Hygiene also has seriously limited the freedom of action of the Commissioner as compared with the freedom accorded the Commissioner of Health. The heads of the Department's institutions traditionally have enjoyed considerable autonomy in their jurisdictions. One official in the governor's office facetiously likened them to "medieval barons" and in the same vein suggested that to make changes "the Commissioner has to call an ecumenical council." Consequently, the commissioners and their immediate subordinates had cause to avoid involvements in the Council that could create strains in the internal cohesion of the Department, which partly explains some of the Department's reluctance to participate in the Council.

On the other hand, the Commissioner has the advantage of being directly responsible to the governor, who appoints him for the length of the gubernatorial term, also with the consent of the state senate, as in the case of the Commissioner of Health. However, this strength was usually employed to delay Council action, as for example, when the Commissioner encouraged the governor to designate the Department of Mental Hygiene as the state agency to plan services for the mentally retarded, rather than to name the Council, as the other members preferred.

The Department of Social Welfare

Although it is the second largest agency, the Department of Social Welfare also tended to view the Council negatively, and thus to emphasize the costs of involvement at the expense of the benefits. A person close to a former commissioner reported that the Commissioner "didn't give a damn about the thing," meaning the Council. However, unlike the negativism of the Department of Mental Hygiene, the attitude of the Department of Social Welfare seems to have been more a reaction to the vigorous behavior of the Department of Health than a temperamental preference to be left alone. The informant already quoted felt that the Commissioner mainly went to Council meetings "in self-defense." Of all the agencies belonging to the Council, the Department of Social Welfare feared the Department of Health most. The head of another department reported that the Commissioner just referred to "really felt that . . . [the Department of Health] wanted to take over everything." As in the case of the Department of Mental Hygiene, the Department of Social Welfare's views of the Council also altered in the later years, but apparently as much a result of changes in the outlook of the Department of Health as a consequence of differences in the character of the agency.

The Department of Social Welfare also worried that its interests might suffer from involvement in the Council. But like the other agencies, it too was successful in blocking all serious attempts to move the Council to confront issues that seemed to threaten its vital interests. Certainly there is no evidence that the Department ever lost anything of value through participation, such as responsibilities and resources. Consequently the Department's past tendency to see value in the Council only as a mechanism for keeping an eye on the other agencies, especially on the Department of Health, seems to have been somewhat dysfunctional for its interests.

The Department of Social Welfare is substantially larger than the Department of Health, when compared by budget size. Even its health budget is somewhat greater. Yet, the Department has a number of serious weaknesses that diminish its strength and that incline it to cautiousness, factors that have contributed to its negative outlook in the Council.

First and foremost, the Department is not a unified agency and tends to reflect an equilibrium of political forces. Authority is divided at the very top between a Board of Social Welfare and the Commissioner, who is not wholly responsible to the governor. In the words of a recent distinguished state commission that studied the Department:

> The present division of policy-making and administrative authority between the State Board of Social Welfare and the State Commissioner creates confusion as to which is responsible for public welfare programs, and which should exert constructive leadership.
>
> The present system also removes the Governor from direct responsibility for welfare operations and sets the State Commissioner apart from the Governor's cabinet. This proves a liability in joint action with the other departments of the State government and in relations with the Federal government.[20]

In 1964, the lines of communication from the Commissioner of Social Welfare to the governor were strengthened, when the law was changed to provide for the Commissioner to be appointed

20. *Public Welfare in the State of New York* (Albany, N. Y., Jan. 15, 1963).

by the Board with the consent of the governor.[21] Previously, the governor's approval had not been required. The Department also is the center of a play of divergent political interests that have profited from the diffusion of organizational power. Some of the most important interests that press upon the Department have become institutionalized in the Board itself. Among those familiar with the Department, it is common knowledge that appointments customarily are divided equally among representatives of Protestant, Catholic, and Jewish welfare interests. Of course, factors other than religious and moral views enter into the formation of state welfare policy, and many groups find a voice in it, such as nonsectarian voluntary health and welfare agencies, and taxpayer associations. However, since the play of interests is broad, and because the groups frequently diverge in outlook, the result tends to be a stalemate. In the opinion of a top official of another Council agency, "Their [the Department's] constituency is interested in their doing nothing."

The Department of Social Welfare also labors under the burden of generally unfavorable public attitudes toward public welfare, which necessarily raises the sensitivity of departmental personnel. Unlike mental health, which traditionally has been pushed out of sight and into the arms of physicians, public welfare is visible, for most services are at the local level where they can be watched. It is everybody's business, as well as that of private charities and religious organizations doing good works. Thus, in public welfare, social attitudes, morality, and the pocketbook converge to produce some of the most heated criticism of the role and effectiveness of government. The general reluctance of the public to support welfare budgets also has kept the Department under constant pressure, such as that from taxpayer groups to insure that the government isn't cheated. This has resulted in a heavy emphasis in welfare administration upon determining the financial eligibility of clients, with its concomitant red tape, at the expense of the recipients' rehabilitation. Much of the criticism of public welfare

21. *New York Laws of 1964*, Chap. 281, Sec. 3.

has had the quality of a self-fulfilling prophecy. Most welfare assistance also goes to minority groups, which does not improve the public standing of welfare programs. Moreover, being unorganized, the poor have been unable to provide the Department of Social Welfare with any meaningful political support, except as they are represented by surrogate groups, which have their own ideas about helping the underprivileged. Thus, while the Department is highly attuned to political realities, it has much difficulty in controlling its own destiny. It is not certain, in fact, of its central role or of how it is expected to function.

The Department of Social Welfare also suffers from a "lack of professional cement," which inhibits its cohesiveness and complicates the problems of its representatives in dealing with other agencies. Although the Department tends to have a social work orientation, few of its personnel are trained social workers, as defined by the profession. Although many persons handling caseloads in welfare agencies consider themselves social workers, only a very small percentage have had formal training in the field. Furthermore, social workers do not receive the recognition and status accorded physicians and educators, who formed the backbone of the other Council agencies. The slowness of the Department to professionalize itself is evident in the custom throughout most of the state, which only recently has been abandoned, of electing local welfare commissioners who, one informant reported, were "hack politicians getting their rewards."[22]

Because of the liabilities just described, Commissioners of Social Welfare and their staffs had to be especially circumspect in their behavior on the Council. Yet, this situation tended to make the typical Commissioner of Welfare of two minds. On the one hand, as the head of an agency subject to the pressures of a complex of interest groups, he had to consider carefully the implications of cooperating with agencies on the Council. On the other hand, as

22. In 1965, the legislature provided for the appointment of such officials by local authorities, effective January 1, 1966. See *New York Laws of 1965*, Chap. 1071, Sec. 1.

a representative of an agency in need of political support, he was inclined to regard the Council as a potential source of such support. Consequently, while the Department of Social Welfare was more interested in the Council than the Department of Mental Hygiene, it was more prone to be frightened away by the Department of Health. However, the Department's attitude toward the Council became more favorable as the pressure on the Council from the Department of Health diminished. The immediate cause of the Department's sensitivity was removed, if not the sensitivity itself.

The State Education Department

Of all the member agencies, the State Education Department had the most composed attitude toward the Council. As the largest and most secure of the departments, it tended to be the Council's balance wheel. An official of another agency, in commenting upon the attitudes of the Departments of Social Welfare and Mental Hygiene and the Education Department toward continuation of the Council in 1960, when its future was uncertain, said that the Commissioner of Education "probably was the only one who felt an intellectual need for this sort of thing." Also, the behavior of the Education Department was more ambivalent than that of the member agencies. More than any of the others, it was inclined to speak with several voices. At the summit, Commissioners of Education tended to assume an above-the-battle point of view, whereas at the committee level, the heads of the Department's health programs had differing attitudes toward the Council. The leaders of one major unit tended to emphasize the advantages of cooperating with the other agencies, whereas the staffs of other units focused largely on the disadvantages and ranged in outlook from cautiousness to outright defensiveness. The response of the Department, more than that of any of the other agencies, was pluralistic. Each of its constituent units that participated in the Council tended to determine its own behavior. The behavior of the Department as a whole, therefore, was not informed by a calculated strategy.

Commissioners of Education were inclined neither to expect more from the Council than it produced nor to fear that their agency's interests would suffer from participation. The same cannot be said of most of the units of the Department that were involved in the Council, however, such as those concerned with school health services and special services to handicapped children. With the exception of the Division of Vocational Rehabilitation, most of the units performing health functions tended to focus on the costs of involvement rather than the benefits. The negative response of these units was encouraged by the efforts of the Department of Health to expand its functions, especially to assume some of the units' responsibilities. Their sensitivity in this respect was of long standing because of the issues involving the possible transfer of functions to the Department of Health that had been brought before the Council. Those involving functions administered by units within the Department of Education had been among the first that the Department of Health urged the Council to consider. A top official of the Education Department acknowledged that many of the agency's staff "were very suspicious of Health."

As in the case of the other agencies, the negative reaction to the Council of the constituent units of the Education Department also seems to have been excessive. Actually these units were quite able to defend themselves because of the ease with which any member could thwart Council action that it felt was antithetical to its interests. There are indications, however, that on some occasions Commissioners of Education were sympathetic to the proposals of the Department of Health and might have assented to them had not their lieutenants disagreed.

Two principal factors contributed to the outlook and behavior of the State Education Department within the Council: the unusual security of the agency, and the character and relative autonomy of its constituent units.

Not only is the Education Department by far the largest agency of state government, but traditionally it has also enjoyed the special independent status frequently accorded public education agencies in the United States. In keeping with the typical

American belief in separating public education from "politics," the Department is somewhat insulated from gubernatorial and other partisan influences, for it is headed by a powerful independent Board of Regents, which has unusually direct access to the legislature. The Commissioner therefore is directly responsible to the Board, which appoints him, and he serves at its pleasure. However, unlike the Board of Social Welfare, which is a nucleus of interest groups, the Board of Regents serves to insulate the Department from some of the usual political pressures that play upon state departments. And, of course, this arrangement also gives preference to others, mainly professional groups in the field of education. The high public esteem accorded education and its heavily professionalized atmosphere also add to the security and separateness of the Department.

The relative independence of the constituent units of the Education Department probably contributed most to the plurality of its voices in the Council. In the words of an official of an agency accustomed to strong central control, "the Department operates very much like a University." Yet, although the authority of the Commissioner is limited, he enjoys high prestige, much as a university president. In fact, the Commissioner of Education is also President of The University of the State of New York.[23] That he is not expected to govern like a monarch, however, is not always understood outside of the Department. An official of another department felt that the Commissioner of Education was "not master in his own house." The autonomy of the Department's units also is reinforced by the highly professional character of its staff. A top representative of the Department was of the opinion that the Department "couldn't get good people if they didn't have freedom."

Consequently, the freedom possessed by the Commissioner of Education to make commitments for his Department in the Council was severely circumscribed. Yet, paradoxically, because of the unusual security of the Department and its collegial atmosphere,

23. The State University of New York is a corporate entity within The University of the State of New York.

the Commissioner, much like the members of his staff, was able to speak out more freely than some of the other commissioners. In a sense, the character of the Department inclined the Commissioner toward an olympian posture. Usually he could count on his units to defend themselves against outsiders as well as to resist his direction when they disagreed with him. For example, it was reported by several members of the Department of Health that some years ago, when the Commissioner of Health approached the Commissioner of Education about the possible transfer of a particular medical function from Education to Health, the Commissioner of Education agreed to support the move provided the Department of Health could convince his deputies to go along with it. The posture of the Commissioner of Education is not without its embarrassment, however, for the difficulties he faces in exercising his authority are easily revealed. Department of Health representatives have indicated that on several occasions understandings between the Commissioners of the two Departments have fallen through because of resistance in the ranks of the Education Department. The enormous size of the Education Department also handicapped the Commissioner in controlling the behavior of his staff in the Council. One of his deputies acknowledged, "It is impossible for the Commissioner to be informed and effective in all areas, because of the size and structure of the Department."

It is difficult to generalize about the factors that shaped the behavior of each of the constituent units of the Education Department in the Council, for each unit tends to have its own character. Nor is it necessary for the purposes at hand to go into such detail. Suffice it to say that the separateness and overall security of the Department have produced an insularity of outlook in many quarters of the agency, which hardly encourages interdepartmental cooperation. However, some of these attitudes have begun to wear away as they have in the other agencies, partly because of the decline in the assertiveness of the Department of Health, and partly because of the changing character of the Education Department's programs.

CHAPTER 5

Council Rules, Strategies, and Processes

SINCE the members of the Council were competitors as well as colleagues, beneath the informality of their deliberations lay the potential danger that fundamental disagreements might break through and disrupt proceedings. Sometimes this danger was close at hand as a result of the perseverance and skill with which the Department of Health tried, albeit unsuccessfully, to steer Council action on controversial issues. But codes of appropriate behavior, which insure the cohesiveness of a group and permit it to function, developed in the Council, as they invariably do in all continuing groups.[1] In fact, one of the main functions of these norms of behavior was to protect the members from direct conflict. Yet, although the Council eschewed controversial issues, the struggle among the members to advance their views certainly did not cease; rather, divergent views took restrained and tolerable forms. An understanding of how the Council operated, therefore, demands elucidation of the norms and practices that guided the behavior of the members.[2]

1. For a full treatment of the development and functions of norms in groups, see the classic work by George C. Homans, *The Human Group* (New York, 1950), esp. pp. 121–27.

2. Peter M. Blau and W. Richard Scott point out that: "It is impossible to understand the nature of a formal organization without investigating the networks of informal relations and the unofficial norms as well as the for-

It will therefore be instructive to investigate (1) the most important rules that governed the conduct of the members; (2) the principal strategies and tactics that were employed by the agencies to advance and defend their views of the public interest and thus their maintenance needs; and (3) the processes by which the Council operated.

Council rules and practices reflected the advantages and disadvantages that induced the Council members to cooperate. They emerged from the dynamics of Council activity and from the vital interests of the members, in contrast to being imposed by higher authority. During the entire life of the Council, the governor and the legislature conspicuously left it to the members to work out their own ground rules.

No norms can ever be adhered to completely, a truth recognized in all human organizations. But Council rules were observed by the members with remarkable fidelity. Moreover, on the occasions when any individual member attempted to override them, they usually prevailed.

Furthermore, in the vying for advantage, which proceeds by various strategies and tactics, the defender clearly had the better part of any struggle, for use of stratagems was circumscribed by rules that protected the interests of each member from any serious threat.

The Council operated by analytic rather than bargaining processes, that is, through such means as persuasion and problem-solving, with heavy emphasis upon the exchange of information and fact-finding studies.[3] Since no bargaining occurred within the Council, this is further evidence that it was not a mechanism for the direct management of conflict among its members, bar-

mal hierarchy of authority and the official body of rules." See *Formal Organizations* (San Francisco, 1962), p. 6.

3. The distinction employed was advanced by James G. March and Herbert A. Simon, who classify problem-solving and persuasion as analytic processes and bargaining and politics as bargaining processes. See *Organizations* (New York, 1958), pp. 112–35.

gaining being the usual way in which organizations settle their differences.[4]

Rules of the Game

The most important Council rules, those of primary concern here, were informal.[5] The Council also had written bylaws dating from 1956, which were prepared by the staff, but these mainly reaffirmed the Council's purposes and delineated in broad terms the formal responsibilities of committees and staff.

Without doubt, the most important Council rule was that all decisions were to be made by unanimous agreement, for observance of this norm was a primary means by which the members avoided controversial issues. Therefore, the Council almost never voted, except to confirm a consensus. An official who participated in Council committees for many years reported, "There's practically no formal voting . . . most things never come up for a vote . . . it's not the kind of business that you vote on."

The number of instances in which a divided vote occurred can be counted on one hand, as a review of the minutes reveals. Each of these involved a situation in which the Council was unable to avoid a controversial issue. Moreover, most of these divisions of opinion took place at the committee level, and the issues usually were rejected by the Council as a whole.

One instance occurred very early in the history of the Council when it was considering methods of improving health services to school children through coordination of the efforts of public health and education officials, particularly efforts at the local level. The problem had been brought up mainly at the urging of the Department of Health, which believed strongly that school health functions should be transferred from educational to public

4. *Ibid.*

5. These rules seemed mainly to have had latent, or unintended and unrecognized, functions as compared with manifest, or intended, functions. See Robert K. Merton, *Social Theory and Social Structure* (rev. ed.; New York, 1957), pp. 19–84.

health officials. It also was one of several questions suggested in Governor Dewey's directive creating the Council (which the Department of Health had helped to prepare)[6] as requiring Council attention. The difficulties began when the Department vigorously pressed its views in the committee that had been established to consider the problem. At one point the Department of Health was so resolute that the committee was unable to agree on how to implement recommendations for coordinating public health and school health services. The chairman of the committee, who was a representative of the Department of Health, insisted on proposing to the Council that it encourage local school districts to arrange with local health officials to provide school health services.[7] But since they were utterly unwilling to consider any diminution of their responsibilities, the representatives of the Education Department strenuously opposed the proposal. This impasse split the committe down the middle, with Mental Hygiene voting with Health and Social Welfare lining up with Education. This situation was one of the rare instances in which members other than the immediate contestants entered a fray. Having been pushed to take a position, the opposition was unusually frank in making known its objections to the chairman's proposal: "The education authorities would be giving up their authority or turning over their responsibilities to the Health Department."[8]

After avoiding the issue for over a year and a half, the Council finally rejected the controversy. It "agreed that the Committee be asked to reconsider this recommendation, and, if those members who voted in favor of its inclusion still wish it to be included in the report, that it appear separately as a minority report recommendation."[9] Although the point in dispute was

6. See pp. 24–27.

7. Recommendations from Sub-Committee on Coordination of School and Community Health Services, July, 1948. Exhibit 4, attached to the Agenda, IHC meeting, Feb. 1, 1950.

8. The opposition also gave as a secondary reason: "[Private] physicians would be in open opposition because they would consider the Health Department intruding into the practice of medicine" (*ibid.*, p. 4).

9. Minutes of the IHC, Feb. 1, 1950, p. 4.

dropped from future reports, the issue was never resolved; it was dropped instead. The continued existence of the disagreement was acknowledged more than five years later when, in the winter of 1953, the Council accepted the committee's own recommendation that it be discontinued and that the Departments of Education and Health pick up the remaining threads. In the words of the committee chairman, the controversial proposal was "the only recommendation of the Committee's work which had not been approved unanimously."[10]

On another occasion, a member abstained rather than be registered in opposition to his colleagues. In this instance, the Commissioners of Health and Mental Hygiene felt strongly that the Council should reaffirm its opposition to the licensing of chiropractors, which for years it unanimously had opposed. But, reversing itself, the Board of Regents of the State Education Department had come out in support of the impending legislation, which tied the hands of the Commissioner of Education. Thus, rather than oppose his colleagues, the Commissioner of Education abstained when the Council again voted to oppose the licensing of chiropractors.[11] This also was one of the few times that a Council recommendation was made to the governor without unanimity. Obviously, there was considerable regret among the members. As one commissioner reported about a similar instance of open disagreement, in which a formal vote was not taken, "It worried the [Council] that it couldn't present a united point of view to the [governor's staff]."

In one instance the Council accepted a majority report of one of its committees after months of futile efforts to achieve unanimity; later the Council issued the report as a public document. This unusual occurrence involved the Council's Advisory Committee on Nursing Services, which was formed in 1949 to study the severe shortage of nurses that followed World War II, and which, two years later, made innovative proposals for the improvement of

10. *Ibid.*, Nov. 24, 1953, p. 7.
11. Minutes of the IHHC, Feb. 28, 1961, pp. 8–9.

nursing education and service.[12] Unlike other committees, this advisory group included several private citizens who represented the nursing profession, as well as personnel of the member agencies. The willingness of the Council to choose up sides in this instance can be explained by the fact that one of the dissenters was a private member and the other was outvoted by two other representatives of his own agency, the State Education Department. Thus, the Commissioner of Education had the principal burden of decision.

A corollary of the rule of unanimity was the custom of "senatorial courtesy." The Council would not take action on a question, if, in exploring the matter, it was found that one or several members were strongly opposed. Accordingly, the Commissioner of Mental Hygiene was able to forestall consideration of the issue over which state agency should be assigned responsibility for planning services for the mentally retarded, even though the other members were very anxious to discuss it. In other words, a majority was not willing to impose its will on a minority. As one commissioner said, "This is verboten." Although it sometimes encouraged voting, the Department of Health "knew it couldn't force its ideas on others," as one of the Department's representatives acknowledged.

It still remains to be explained why the rule of unanimity was so sacrosanct. The answer is that the costs of conflict were too high. For the Council to operate by majority rule would enable the members to form coalitions and thus coercive factions. This would threaten the vital interests of the agencies and intensify the competition among them. The taking of sides would have reduced the element of predictability in members' relations, and thus would have made cooperation extremely difficult, even when it was desirable; as for example, in influencing groups in their external environment and in developing relationships among their programs. Although some Council members keenly would have liked to acquire certain functions assigned to others, a common interest

12. *Proposal for the Improvement of Nursing Education and Service* (Albany, N. Y., Dec. 1950).

in self-preservation prevailed over any desire for majority rule with its attendant risks.[13]

To repeat a central factor, even if the members found it beneficial to run the risks of majority rule, there was no way in which the Council could implement its decisions. Since it lacked any legal authority and could impose no sanctions, the Council had to depend upon the voluntary compliance of its members. Nor could the Council count on the governor and the legislature for backing. The members also fully appreciated that each of them had access to the governor, and could thus appeal "over the head" of the Council when its interests were at stake. Furthermore, each of the agencies had a constituency that could be mobilized to assist in defense of its interests and, equally important, one that probably could not be kept out of a battle, once it started. With the possibilities that conflict might spread, there also was danger that the agencies might lose control of the situation.

The rule of unanimity really reflected an unwritten understanding that it was improper for a member to bring up matters involving basic conflict, a fact well illustrated by an instance in which one agency ignored the rule. As related by an official who witnessed the incident:

> The Commissioner of Department A had been sniping at [an issue involving Department B] . . . for some time. . . . [On this occasion] he decided to launch a full-scale attack when the Commissioner of

13. Arthur J. Vidich and Joseph Bensman, in their study *Small Town in Mass Society* (New York, 1960), found that the rule of unanimity, which prevailed in a village board, also served the function of avoiding controversy: "Beneath the public unanimity of the board, there exist small but important differences of interest between board members. . . . Yet this conflict is never openly apparent and the principle of unanimity of decision is never broken" (p. 129). They also found that the board relies heavily upon discussion in order to find consensus, much as the Council does. However, in contrast to the Council, the basic reasons for unanimity in the board lay beyond the immediate interests of the members. Mainly, unanimity served to protect the dominance in decision-making of the political machine on which the board members were utterly dependent in the performance of their official roles.

> Department B was in the chair and had to take it. The others came to the defense of the Commissioner of B. . . . The Commissioner of A not only infuriated the Commissioner of B, but his power play polarized the others.

According to this informant, the other agencies came to the defense of the beleaguered department, not because the criticism of Commissioner B's program was invalid, but because it violated the unwritten understanding that one agency doesn't embarrass another by bringing up basic disagreements, at least directly. The underlying significance of this norm was clearly revealed by the informant when he explained that behind the others' defense of the Commissioner of Department B was the feeling that "today it is the Commissioner of Department B, tomorrow it may be us."

Although Council discussions were very informal, the members usually did not participate in decisions unless their interests were involved. This was particularly true when there was any disagreement. One of the commissioners commented that agencies whose interests were not at stake were "not in a position to choose sides" during moments of controversy. In such cases it was almost axiomatic that the parties to the dispute would be asked to settle the issue privately, if they themselves did not suggest it, a move which permanently removed the source of disagreement to another arena, at least in most instances. Thus, for example, at the end of the IHRB period, the Council concurred with the suggestion of the Commissioner of Mental Hygiene that the Departments of Health and Mental Hygiene should work out their differences over disposition of the Council's alcoholism program. Moreover, it was tacitly understood that a controversial question usually would not be brought up again, unless the members directly concerned requested it.

In addition to avoiding the unpleasantness of becoming embroiled in disagreements, Council members felt that there was little or no advantage in participating in decisions that did not affect their interests. To become involved would mean at the very least to run the risk of displeasing some, if not all, of the interested parties. The practice that only the interested could take part in decisions, except those decisions that predictably would make a consensus unanimous, had the latent consequence of reducing the number of agencies that might be in disagreement. Depending upon the degree of disagreement, it also helped to isolate the source of friction, as in the example cited above.

It was customary for the agency with the largest stake in a question under consideration to be given the leadership in studying it and presenting it for discussion. This was most evident in the choice of committee chairmen. Even though the Council customarily rotated the chairmanships of the most active committees among its core members, usually the agency with a predominant stake in a committee's activities was favored, at least initially.[14] To illustrate: a representative of the Department of Insurance was made chairman of the committee established to develop proposals to encourage the underwriting of insurance covering the cost of catastrophic illness. Similarly, representatives of the Department of Mental Hygiene chaired the committees on mental retardation, emotionally disturbed children, alcoholism, and narcotics addiction when they were reformed after reorganization of the Council early in the Rockefeller administration. The Department of Mental Hygiene also chaired these committees for a longer time than any other department. The practice of conferring the lead on the most interested agency further insured that the vital interests of the members with the most to lose would be adequately protected. Paradoxically, the practice also was dysfunctional when the leading agency asked the other members to discuss matters they preferred to avoid, as for example, when the Department of Health chaired the Committees on School Health and Rehabilitation and called on other members for comment on controversial issues.

In conclusion, the informal rules of the Council effectively discouraged competition among the agencies from invading the

14. This was true during the IHC and the IHHC periods. During the IHRB phase, the Executive Director chaired all Council committees.

mechanism. Consequently, they made it possible for the members to reap many of the benefits of cooperating when their interests were not in fundamental conflict. Moreover, the rules were remarkably strong, as was demonstrated by their capacity to contain an assertive member. Council norms, particularly the rule of unanimity, also helped to assure the survival of the Council.[15] In the absence of sanctions or strong outside pressures that could compel cooperation, all evidence suggests that the Council could not tolerate much conflict.

Strategies and Tactics

Although Council rules assured the members considerable predictability, and thus security, in their relations they did not remove the struggle for advantage. Instead they channeled its pursuit into acceptable and tolerable forms. The members employed a variety of strategies and tactics to advance their aims and to defend themselves against actions that they felt might be injurious. However, the sparring was gentlemanly and favored the defense, for it was circumscribed by the rules of the game. Consequently, except for an occasional tense moment, Council deliberations were generally relaxed and informal.

The strategies and tactics are described here primarily in terms of their intent and effect as offensive and defensive maneuvers. Although a military analogy is used, the strategies themselves are regarded as neutral. Moreover, there is no implication that in employing strategies to pursue their interests the agencies did not act in the public interest as they saw it. On the contrary, they necessarily had to engage in offensive and defensive as well as cooperative behavior because of the inevitable differences in their maintenance needs and in their views of the public interest. This

15. Edward C. Banfield found that civic associations, including the Welfare Council, that played a part in the six cases he studied of decision-making in Chicago "avoided controversy in order to maintain themselves." See *Political Influence* (New York, 1961), pp. 297–99.

may seem anomalous to some because, as Leonard Sayles has observed:

Most Americans and Western Europeans are brought up to believe that consensus and unity are an essential ingredient for any successful political, social, or economic institution. But this belief in oneness does not square with the facts.[16]

Actually, as Lewis Coser has pointed out:

Groups require disharmony as well as harmony, disassociation as well as association; and conflicts within them are by no means altogether disruptive factors. . . . Conflict as well as co-operation has social functions. Far from being necessarily dysfunctional, a certain degree of conflict is an essential element in group formation and the persistence of group life.[17]

Offensive Strategies and Tactics

The Department of Health made the most effective use of strategies and tactics for offensive purposes. During the period when it was vigorously pursuing its interests, the cornerstone of the Department's strategy was to maintain the initiative vis-à-vis the other agencies, as described in Chapter 4. Mainly, the Department of Health attempted to introduce many items on the

16. Leonard R. Sayles, *Managerial Behavior* (New York, 1964) pp. 140–41.

17. Lewis A. Coser, *The Functions of Social Conflict* (New York, 1956), p. 31. Coser also explains why organization members tend not to recognize the value of conflict: "The decision-makers are engaged in maintaining, and, if possible, strengthening the organizational structures through and in which they exercise power and influence. Whatever conflicts occur within these structures will appear to them to be dysfunctional. Firmly wedded to the existing order by interest and sentiment, the decision-maker tends to view departures from this order as the result of psychological malfunctioning. . . . He will, therefore, be more likely to concern himself with 'tensions' or with 'stresses' and 'strains' than with other aspects of conflict behavior that might indicate pressures for changing basic institutional arrangements. Also, decision-makers are more likely to consider the dysfunctions of conflict for the total structure, without giving attention to the functions of conflict for particular groups or strata within it" (pp. 27–28).

agenda in the expectation that some would be decided to its advantage or would have ramifications outside the Council that would work in its favor. Consequently, the role of the Department in the selection of Council business overshadowed that of all the other agencies. For example, as has been indicated, the Department directly initiated 56 percent of all the rehabilitation issues that were first raised by the members (20 of 36). However, not only did the Department of Health raise more agenda items than any other members, but even more importantly, it brought up most of the controversial issues. For instance, it was directly responsible for bringing up 71 percent of the controversial rehabilitation issues initiated by the member agencies (5 of 7). Furthermore, the Department ably employed most of the available tactics both to raise such issues and to press their consideration. Yet, although it was the most energetic and skillful strategist in this respect, the Department of Health was not the only member to employ tactics for offensive purposes.

Encouraging studies. One of the most effective ways of bringing a delicate question to the Council's attention was to recommend that the matter be studied. It is difficult to object to a study, since the very process implies objectivity and suspended judgment. Moreover, all of the interested parties may be assured representation on the study team, which helps to disarm any opposition. Of special advantage, a study draws attention to the very questions that its initiator may have in mind. Further, the study process also tends to raise other questions on which it may be possible to capitalize.

Most of the agencies suggested studies at some time, but the Department of Health did so more often in order to raise controversial questions. As an example: In the fall of 1954, the Commissioner of Health called for a study of the state's responsibilities for the supervision of hospitals, saying that "perhaps the time has come when the whole field of hospital care should be considered and departmental activities synchronized in such a way as to avoid duplication of activities."[18] In bringing up this ques-

18. Minutes of the IHC, Sept. 28, 1954, p. 4.

tion, the Commissioner of Health touched upon an extremely sensitive issue, the disagreement over which agency—his Department or the Department of Social Welfare—should have state responsibilities for the inspection of hospitals. By calling for a study that was perfectly reasonable, and which brought up the issue tangentially, he hoped to gain support for his agency's belief that it logically should be assigned the hospital functions of the Department of Social Welfare. The outcome was the creation of a committee that was short-lived and that successfully evaded the underlying conflict.

Creating a committee. A corollary tactic, one also employed in the instance just described, is to recommend or encourage the creation of a special or, probably better still, a standing committee. A committee provides a continuing vehicle for raising issues and generating studies, and thus increases an agency's opportunity to bring up questions that may be to its advantage to have considered. For example, the Department of Health sought creation of the Committee on Rehabilitation in 1953, at least in part, because it believed that such a committee might help convince the other members that the medical functions of the Division of Vocational Rehabilitation would be upgraded if they were supervised by the Health Department's medical staff. Thus, during the Council discussions of the agencies' rehabilitation programs that preceded the decision to establish the Committee, the Commissioner of Health suggested, "A committee of the Council will be indicated when the discussions have been concluded."[19]

Defining issues in acceptable terms. Another tactic that the departments used to advance potentially controversial aims was to define the issues they wished to press in terms that were calculatedly acceptable to other members. This maneuver, if successful, puts the opposition at some disadvantage by making objection philosophically and semantically difficult. The Department of Health employed this tactic several times in hopes that the Committee on Rehabilitation would consider the transfer of certain medical responsibilities of the other agencies to its own aegis. For

19. *Ibid.*, Feb. 24, 1953, p. 7.

example, in one such instance the Department of Health defined the issue as broadly as possible. In commenting on the new activities of his department in the field of chronic illness, the Commissioner of Health suggested that the Council and its Committee on Rehabilitation concentrate on the definition of the problems of chronic disease in their broadest sense:

> The Committee on Rehabilitation should be requested to consider the constitutional responsibilities of the respective departments in this field. . . . An analysis such as this would facilitate the development of recommendations for a State-wide program outlining the departmental functions and responsibilities and those functions which should be carried out on an interdepartmental basis.[20]

Masking conflict in noncontroversial terms. Since it was a violation of the rules to bring up issues that involved basic conflict, one way of evading the rules to some extent was to mask such issues in noncontroversial terms. This tactic, which is a variant of defining issues in acceptable terms, was used in 1954 by the Department of Health when it recommended that the Council "review the responsibilities of each department in the hospital program of the State, including the current activities of each department and the staff which each has to carry out in its activities."[21] There was no suggestion that the Committee on Hospitals, which the members agreed to establish, should consider the possible transfer of responsibilities from one department to another. It is highly doubtful that the other agencies would have agreed to set up a committee if the Commissioner of Health had made such a suggestion. Yet, underlying the request was the hope that the raising of the hospital issue would help to show that the Department of Health was better qualified than the Department of Social Welfare to carry out the state's responsibilities for inspection of hospitals.

Invoking outside pressure. On some occasions a Council member encouraged the governor or a powerful interest group to

20. *Ibid.*, March 23, 1954, p. 2.
21. *Ibid.*, Sept. 28, 1954, p. 5.

request that the Council consider a question that it wished to press. The main advantage of this tactic was that it put pressure on the Council, and thus increased the likelihood that the members would face up to the issue in question. To illustrate: At one time the Departments of Health and Insurance persuaded the governor to support their recommendation that the Council consider the report of a study which they had sponsored dealing with prepayment of medical and hospital care.[22] In replying to their suggestion the governor wrote: "I welcome your recommendation that the report be referred to the . . . [Council] for its overall consideration. Inasmuch as you are members of the Council, I ask that you take appropriate steps to present this report to the Council for such action."[23]

Supported by this missive, the heads of the two departments suggested "that a Committee on Medical Care composed of high level staff members of each department should be appointed to study the Trussell Report as a first assignment and to consider other medical care issues on an outgoing basis."[24] In due course, such a committee was established. The maneuver not only opened up a question that the two departments were anxious to have considered, but it provided the Department of Health with another forum in which it could present its case for leadership in the hospital and medical care field. This stratagem, however, seems not to have been tried often. On the one hand, it was difficult to influence the right parties; on the other, it was likely to annoy the other members if they preferred to avoid the issue in question.

Defensive Strategies and Tactics

Having been anxious to avoid consideration of issues raised by the Department of Health that might lead to any diminution of their functions, the other members pioneered the use of defensive

22. *Prepayment for Medical and Dental Care in New York State,* submitted by School of Public Health and Administrative Medicine, Columbia University, to Hon. Herman E. Hilleboe, Commissioner of Health, and Hon. Thomas Thacher, Superintendent of Insurance, Oct. 1962.

23. Letter from Governor Nelson A. Rockefeller to Dr. Herman E. Hilleboe and the Hon. Thomas Thacher, IHHC, Albany, Oct. 12, 1962.

24. Minutes of the IHHC, Oct. 23, 1962, p. 3.

strategies and tactics. This was particularly true of the Departments of Mental Hygiene and Social Welfare, for they felt most threatened by the attempts of the Department of Health to bring up controversial matters, as was discussed in Chapter 4. Yet, it is an exaggeration to say that the behavior of the other agencies was influenced by a strategy. Their actions seem to have been guided more by a wariness, a desire to avoid involvements that might endanger their interests, than by clear objectives and a conscious plan of action. Consequently, the other agencies were cautious not to bring up agenda items that another member could exploit at their expense.

Listening politely. Perhaps the most common technique that the agencies used to resist each other's sallies was to ignore them. By politely listening to offending recommendations and not responding, or by responding innocuously, members of the Council often averted decisions they wished to avoid. For example, on one occasion, believing that the Department of Health was seeking an opportunity to present its case for performing some of their rehabilitation functions, the other members failed to act on the suggestion of the Commissioner of Health "that the people experienced in the field of rehabilitation in each department should be asked to review the resources available in the other departments to see whether they can make use of these services and whether there can be more effective mutual assistance."[25] In effect, the other agencies interpreted the recommendation as a matter not requiring action and thus avoided the issue. The virtue of this tactic is that it usually forces the initiator either to let the matter drop or to show his hand. Obviously, if he should choose the latter course, he runs the risk of violating the rules of the game as well as being defeated.

Stalling. Stalling was an equally effective and commonly practiced technique for averting unfavorable action. It also has many variations, including: asking that a question be tabled; taking excessive time in following through on a commitment; and asking

25. Minutes of the IHRB, May 27, 1958, p. 7.

that a matter be restudied. The object of stalling is to beg time to get countermeasures underway, or, if these are not possible, to allow time for the situation to change. When in 1963 the other agencies were anxious to discuss the question of which state agency should be given responsibility for mental retardation planning, the Commissioner of Mental Hygiene repeatedly stalled, employing various excuses. Once, after a committee of the Council had come out in favor of the Council doing the planning, he requested that action on the Committee's recommendation "be deferred until specific [federal] legislation is passed."[26] In the meantime his Department was preparing the state's application for a federal planning grant. The instance in which the Commissioner of Social Welfare asked for clarification of Governor Rockefeller's request that the Council assist in the development of a model nursing-home code is another good example of stalling. The Department of Mental Hygiene also used this tactic when the Council was considering the suggestions of its staff for the transfer of the Council's demonstration projects to the member agencies. The Commissioner of Mental Hygiene's request for committee review of the recommendation calling for transfer of the alcoholism project to the Department of Health was a stall, for he accepted without question all of the proposals for the transfer of responsibilities to his own Department.

Not implementing agreements. A last-ditch tactic for avoiding undesirable action, which seldom was used, was to block implementation of Council agreements. This practice, akin to stalling, was rarely necessary, as the rules almost invariably protected the members from having to accept decisions to which they were strongly opposed. For obvious reasons, not following through is a costly tactic that can boomerang. Apparently, this strategem was used by the Department of Mental Hygiene during the episode in which the Council had difficulty agreeing on what steps should be taken to improve state services for emotionally disturbed blind children. Although it had reluctantly agreed to

26. Minutes of the IHHC, July 8, 1963, p. 4.

expand its services to these children, the Department of Mental Hygiene failed to request funds in its next budget to implement the Council's decision. When, at a joint meeting of the Council and the Governor's Council on Rehabilitation, it was suggested that state budget officials were at fault for not earmarking the necessary funds, the representative of the Division of the Budget protested "that no previous budget request for this service had been submitted."[27] Only then did the Department of Mental Hygiene follow through.

Taking Advantage of the Council's Structure

The members also took advantage of the structure of the Council for both offensive and defensive purposes. For example, when individual member agencies held the chairmanship, they used the office to stimulate the flow of agenda items, guide discussions at meetings to ward off threatening issues, and interpret Council decisions to committees and others. On one notable occasion the staffing of the Council also was the source of keen competition for advantage. Even the organization of the Council at times caused strife because of its strategic and tactical importance. In struggles to exploit the structure of the Council, the Department of Health had the upper hand, but never to the extent of abrogating the rules of the game.

Use of the chairmanship. The tactical use of the chairmanship, which was seldom obtrusive, was helpful in influencing the selection of Council business, formally as well as informally. Not only did the chairman possess the advantages of officiating at meetings, but he also oversaw the preparation of the agenda. It was customary for the staff to prepare a proposed agenda, based upon their anticipation of appropriate issues as well as upon the requests of the members, which then was submitted to the chairman for approval. Although, according to the three persons who headed the staff during the life of the Council, chairmen usually agreed

27. Minutes of Joint Meeting of the Governor's Council on Rehabilitation and the IHHC, May 29, 1961, p. 3.

with the staff suggestions, they nonetheless subtly influenced the choice of agenda items. Mainly, chairmen sometimes used their position to add new items, define the issues at hand, or postpone a question. But equally important, the right of the chairman to approve the agenda necessarily influenced to some extent the items that the staff have proposed.[28]

The Department of Health benefited most from the tactical value of the chairmanship, mainly because of its favored position in the organization of the Council. The Commissioner of Health was the chairman, ex officio, through the first decade, that is, the IHC period, 1946–1956, which contributed a great deal to the Department's ability to influence the agenda. The chairmanship of the Council was also of greater value to the Department of Health because the position was better suited to implementing a positive strategy of raising issues than a negative one of avoiding them. Leadership in the chair was much more acceptable, and harder to object to, than obstructive behavior.

Influencing the choice of staff. There was only one open quarrel among the members over the choice of staff, but it was consequential because of underlying strategic and tactical factors. At the beginning of the IHRB period, 1956–1960, when the Council was elevated to the position of an independent agency, the role of the staff changed from one that was essentially secretarial to one of an executive level. Recognizing that the staff would, as a result, have more influence in the choice of business and in the actions taken by the Council, each of the members was anxious that an executive director be appointed who was as sympathetic as possible to its interests. Thus, the Departments of Social Welfare and Mental Hygiene advanced a highly competent person experienced in the fields of social welfare and mental illness. The Department of Health objected and strongly questioned his qualifications, putting forward its own candidate, an

28. Their behavior may be said to obey Carl Friedrich's "rule of anticipated reactions." See Carl J. Friedrich, *Constitutional Government and Politics* (New York, 1937), pp. 17–18.

unusually able public health officer with experience in the Departments of Health and Social Welfare. The outcome was that the Department of Health vigorously and successfully pushed its candidate, whom the other members felt was professionally sympathetic to that Department's point of view on many of the key issues dividing the agencies. Although it is difficult to render an objective judgment on how great a tactical advantage the Department of Health gained from its victory, the other members have admittedly felt that it aided the Department in putting pressure on them. This feeling was reflected in the remarks, made late in the IHHC period, of one of the commissioners, who said, "The Board [Council] was more closely related to the Health Department than it is now."

Reorganization of the council. The Department of Health on a number of occasions put forward proposals for reorganization of the Council to make the mechanism a more effective vehicle for pursuit of its view of the public interest and to reduce the burden of interdepartmental meetings. Primarily it sought, with some success, a broadening of the membership of the Council and, with less success, expansion of the Council's scope through combining it with several other interdepartmental bodies. Thus, the Department of Health played a major part in shaping each of the reorganizations of the Council, including: the increase in its membership in 1953; the further increase in membership and establishment of the Council as an independent agency in 1956; and the saving of the mechanism in 1960, albeit with a reduction in scope, status, and membership. The principal objective and effect of most of these changes from the Department's point of view was to give itself a larger area of operation and thus wider opportunities. Nevertheless, the reorganizations did not alter the Council's informal rules. Since such changes were a product of the Council's relations with the governor and others, they are discussed more fully in the next chapter.

An episode during which the Department of Health pushed the Council about as far as it could is worth relating because it well illustrates various contending tactics and the capacity of the Council to avoid conflict. It took place in the middle 1950's, when the Department of Health hoped the Committee on Rehabilitation would consider the merits of its assertion that it was best qualified to supervise some of the medical functions of the other agencies, particularly those of the Division of Vocational Rehabilitation of the Education Department. Having persuaded his fellow commissioners to ask the Committee to broaden its study of state rehabilitation services, the Commissioner of Health took the opportunity as chairman of the Council to present his Department's case. First he met with the chairman and staff of the Committee, and while conveying the Council's new instructions, suggested that the Committee consider the possible transfer of responsibilities: "This matter [the idea of the medical services of the Vocational Division being supervised or directed by the Health Department] should not be considered as closed."[29] In an unusual charge, he also appealed to the Committee to suspend the rule of unanimity: "When making recommendations, we should not be influenced by apparent difficulties in reorganization. . . . If necessary, majority and minority reports shall be prepared if unanimity of opinion cannot be reached."[30]

Two months later, the Commissioner of Health met personally with the Committee and increased the pressure, apparently feeling that unless he did the other members might stall or avoid the issue. It is reported that he told the Committee:

> Recommendations should be developed for regulations within the departments or for working agreements among the departments to make the best use of available facilities and the services which each department is able to render. For example, the services of vocational counselors or experts in vocational training or placement could be supplied by the Education Department to assist in rehabilitation in the State tuberculosis hospitals [Health Department]. On the other hand, the medical aspects of the rehabilitation program in the Education Department could become a service rendered by the Health

29. Memorandum for the record, April 5, 1954, attached to Minutes of the Committee on Rehabilitation, IHC, April 13, 1954.
30. *Ibid.*

Department. In addition, consideration could also be given to methods of handling the medical rehabilitation problems of the Department of Social Welfare [by the Health Department].[31]

On this occasion, the Commissioner of Health also "stressed the importance of cooperation and trust among the departments to effect such recommendations for changes or reassignments of certain portions of departmental functions."[32] And he assured the Committee that the commissioners "have no preconceived ideas of the particular functions of each department."[33]

This appeal graphically illustrated the necessity of minimizing or ignoring the existence of conflict. If the conflict had not been somewhat masked, discussion of the issue would have been impossible, and therefore it would have been difficult to persuade or at least test one's adversaries. To have approached the question head-on would have meant frank acknowledgement that someone wins and someone loses. In the absence of outside sanctions or pressure that would have compelled cooperation, such an admission would have made any agreement impossible. As it turned out, though all were aware of the underlying disagreement, the Commissioner's appeal produced some discussion of the issue.

But, since the other members were adamant about retaining all of their functions, and thus did not want to argue the merits of the issue, the Committee made no recommendations for the transfer of any responsibilities among the departments. Nor were majority and minority reports made, for the other members simply ignored the appeal of the Commissioner of Health. Even the Department of Health did not insist on a vote, knowing that it would only bring defeat. It was tacitly understood by all that no action taken would be threatening to the vital interests of any member. The rule of unanimity prevailed.

During this period, when the restlessness of the Department of Health probably was at its height, the other members came

31. Minutes of the Committee on Rehabilitation, IHC, May 19, 1954, p. 3.
32. *Ibid.*
33. *Ibid.*

as close as ever in the Council's history to forming a defensive coalition. Feeling a common threat, they acted in unison to protect their interests by evading a decision on the issue. As one of the participants at the time commented: "Ironically, the aggressiveness of the Health Department brought the Committee together, and eventually led to their being tamed."

Tactics Not Employed

The tactics that were not employed by the members are almost as revealing about the Council as those that were, particularly in relation to how it handled conflict. Of greatest significance is the fact that the agencies did not form coalitions and rarely appealed to outside authorities, either for offensive or defensive reasons. The use of coalitions for offensive purposes, as has already been suggested, clearly defies the unwritten rule of unanimity. Even in most of the few instances in which votes were split the Council successfully compromised the differences or put aside the issue.

Coalitions simply were not formed for defensive purposes because they were not necessary. The closest the members ever came to forming a defensive alliance was in the early years of the Committee on Rehabilitation when the Department of Health put substantial pressure upon the Committee. But even in this instance such mutual understanding as the defending members developed was largely tacit and was sufficient to prevent serious examination of the issues in question.

Likewise, individual members rarely turned to outside sources, such as to the governor and the legislature, to put pressure on the Council. The only exceptions were during the infrequent instances that an agency successfully encouraged the governor or others to refer a question to the Council for consideration, such as in the example above. Similarly, individual members did not have to appeal to higher authorities to undo Council decisions that they considered to be inimical. Even on the rare occasions that the Council appealed to the governor to settle differences among its members, this was accomplished with the concurrence of all.

And finally, the members rarely attempted to hamstring the Council by avoiding meetings. The remarkably high attendance of the core members attests to this fact.

Consequently, except for an occasional tense moment, the agencies' use of strategies and tactics was pitched at a relatively low key, for there was little to gain by employing them, which helps to explain why Council meetings were relaxed and informal.

Processes

Examination of the processes by which the Council worked sheds further light on how it operated, especially on how it responded to disagreement. Specifically, such examination reveals that the members did not bargain in the Council, which is a typical process through which many organizations resolve conflict. Rather, it shows that Council members tried to persuade each other. In the words of a former participant, the Council was a "place you can persuade; if you are not successful, it is of no value whatsoever in getting what you want." This example lends further confirmation to the finding that the Council was not a mechanism for resolving conflict.

The following analysis relies heavily upon a discussion of organizational conflict by Herbert Simon and James March, in which they hypothesize that the type of processes employed to resolve conflict is a function of the type of organizational conflict.[34] Identification of the processes by which the Council worked, therefore, is suggestive of the type and amount of conflict it handled. Although their discussion focuses mainly upon conflict within organizations, March and Simon consider their scheme applicable to both inter- and intraorganizational situations.

Their thesis runs as follows: An organization reacts to conflict by two types of processes, analytic and bargaining.[35] In seeking

34. March and Simon, pp. 112–35.

35. March and Simon divide analytic processes into problem-solving and persuasion and bargaining processes into bargaining and politics, but the broader distinction seems adequate.

solutions by means of the first, it is assumed that objectives are shared; if not, emphasis is placed upon gathering information and upon the testing of subgoals for consistency with common objectives. In the case of bargaining, disagreement over goals is taken as fixed and agreement without persuasion is sought. As to its source, intergroup conflict arises from "a positive felt need for joint decision-making and of either a difference in goals or a difference in perceptions of reality or both."[36] Consequently, the more fundamental the conflict, that is, the more it is characterized by sharp and inflexible differences in goals and perceptions of reality, the more it can be settled only through bargaining processes. Although March and Simon also suggest that there is a countertendency within organizations to settle disputes through analytic processes, because bargaining strains an organization's status and power systems, they indicate that there is less pressure for the use of such processes in relations between organizations. Furthermore, they point out that the more organizational conflict is based on intergroup differences, the greater the use of bargaining.[37]

Examination of the way in which the Council functioned reveals no evidence that it served as an instrumentality for bargaining, except indirectly through the isolation and removal of conflict that might be resolved later by the contestants in another arena. At least this was true in the explicit sense, as when one member offered a concession to another in the expectation of reciprocation. By contrast, the Council frequently utilized analytic processes, which further suggests that such conflict as it dealt with did not involve basic differences either in goals or perceptions of reality. In fact, the Council relied heavily upon processes of problem-solving and persuasion, with their accompanying emphasis upon the gathering of data and the exchange of information. Throughout its history the Council and its many ad hoc and continuing

36. March and Simon, p. 121.
37. March and Simon give this as the reason why "the literature on interorganizational conflict has been particularly concerned with the resolution of conflict through bargaining processes—with who gets what" (*ibid.*, p. 131).

committees served as vehicles for the collection and exchange of considerable information and for extended discussion of views. Much of this activity had the latent function of defining areas of agreement and disagreement, and thus of maximizing consensus and isolating conflict that could be resolved only by one member gaining at the expense of another.

There is, however, the further question of whether the members engaged in tacit bargaining in which the "adversaries watch and interpret each other's behavior, each aware that his own actions are being interpreted and anticipated, each acting with a view to the expectations that he creates."[38] This is a difficult question to answer satisfactorily, but it does not seem to apply to the Council, except in the sense that Council deliberations might have changed a member's perceptions of the costs and benefits of a possible decision within the group, and in consequence its behavior, or of a possible course of action outside. Certainly insofar as there was tacit bargaining, it proceeded by analytic processes, which means that it was not bargaining in the sense that March and Simon define it. Furthermore, if there was tacit bargaining it was not bargaining in the sense that "a better bargain for one means less for another,"[39] at least as the agencies themselves perceived

38. Thomas C. Schelling, *The Strategy of Conflict* (Cambridge, Mass., 1963), p. 21. According to Schelling, who defines a bargaining situation as one "in which the ability of one participant to gain his ends is dependent to an important degree on the choices or decisions that the other participant will make," bargaining "may be explicit, as when one offers a concession; or it may be by tacit maneuver, as when one occupies or evacuates strategic territory. It may, as in the ordinary haggling of the market-place, take the *status quo* as its zero point and seek arrangements that yield positive gains to both sides; or it may involve threats of damage, including mutual damage, as in a strike, boycott, or price war, or in extortion" (p. 5).

39. *Ibid.*, p. 21. Schelling also distinguishes between the "efficiency" aspect of bargaining, which "consists of exploring for mutually profitable adjustments," ("For example, can an insurance firm save money, and make a client happier by offering a cash settlement rather than repairing the client's car"), and the "distributional" aspect, which consists of situations "in which a better bargain for one means less for the other." Schelling takes the view that the latter situations "ultimately involve an element of pure bargaining—bargaining in which each party is guided mainly by his expectations of what the other will accept."

the outcome. Such tacit bargaining as may have taken place therefore is indistinguishable from the activities characteristic of the analytic processes that March and Simon describe.

There is no question, however, that attempts by one member to make a gain that might have been at the expense of another member were couched in analytic terms. For example, when the Department of Health sought support for transfer to it of the medical functions of the Division of Vocational Rehabilitation it attempted to persuade the Council that the medical skills and experience of the Department would enable it to provide better services. It, therefore, put its case in terms that the Council could test, if the Council had been disposed to face up to the issue. As a matter of fact, in this unusual episode the Commissioner of Health even seemed willing to bargain, for in his unprecedented and unsuccessful appeal to the Committee on Rehabilitation he suggested a quid pro quo: "The services of vocational counselors or experts in vocational training or placement could be supplied by the Education Department to assist in rehabilitation in the state tuberculosis hospitals,"[40] which were under the jurisdiction of the Department of Health. However, the outcome indicates that the Education Department was not interested in bargaining.

Conflict among organizations can, of course, be settled by recourse to higher authority or by agreement to accept the intervention of a neutral agent either to mediate or to arbitrate disputes. But the instances in which the Council appealed to higher authority to settle an issue were few indeed. The members were loath to present anything but a united front to the governor. Furthermore, there are no instances in which an outside party was consulted, or in which one of the members was called upon, to mediate or arbitrate a dispute. Such practices would have contradicted the informal rules by which the Council operated.

40. Minutes of the Committee on Rehabilitation, IHC, May 19, 1953, p. 3.

CHAPTER 6

Impact of the Environment on the Council

GOVERNORS and, to a much lesser extent, the legislature and private interest groups were the only external groups that were concerned with the Council. Inasmuch as they played a role and influenced the mechanism, they are important to this study of Council operation.[1] Also of interest are the advantages and disadvantages of the Council, from their point of view, including the functions that the mechanism performed for them.

The most salient fact about the behavior of external groups toward the Council is that they left it largely on its own. They seldom attempted to tell the members what questions to consider, and they almost never attempted to manipulate the decision-making process. In fact, none of the governors considered the Council an integral part of his equipment for management of the member agencies. Instead each perceived the mechanism as primarily the agencies' affair.

There were also marked differences in the way each administration valued and supported the Council. Governors Dewey and

1. George C. Homans points out that "an independent enterprise must adapt itself to the environment or go under, but the environment does not dictate an adaptation of any single kind; it only sets limits on the range of adaptations that can take place." See *The Human Group* (New York, 1950), p. 404.

Harriman thought well of the instrumentality and nourished it. They felt that it brought prestige to their administrations and that it was a useful device for coordinating the plans and programs of the member agencies. Furthermore, neither apparently considered it to be a liability in any way. By contrast, Governor Rockefeller and his aides mainly tolerated the Council, and, in the form in which they inherited it (IHRB), they initially perceived it as an impediment to their management of the executive branch. It is likely that the Rockefeller administration would have abolished the mechanism had its members not appealed to the Governor's office, at the urging of the Department of Health. However, with the passage of time the Rockefeller regime became somewhat more favorably disposed to the Council.

The absence of attention to the Council by outside groups, and by governors in particular, profoundly affected its operation. Most important, by permitting the members to control the agenda and the outcome of the decision-making process, they indirectly made it possible for the agencies to avoid controversial issues. Thus governors and others reinforced the Council's inherent aversion to conflict and influenced its character as a decision-making body, including the functions that it performed.[2] The interest of Governors Dewey and Harriman in the mechanism also did much to hold the Council together and encourage the members to cooperate, at least to the extent that their interests were not in basic conflict. Later, the Rockefeller administration's much lower regard and diminished support for the Council weakened the instrumentality and cast it upon uncertain waters.

The Ways in Which External Groups Affected the Council

Governors and others, through action and inaction, influenced the Council's organization, the source and handling of its busi-

2. This raises the question of how the Council would have responded to outside manipulation and how much pressure it could have taken. These questions are discussed in the concluding chapter in considering ways of improving the effectiveness of interdepartmental councils. See Chap. 9.

ness, and the flow of resources and intangible support upon which the mechanism depended for survival. There were also marked differences in the impact of each of the outside forces.

Structure of the Council

All three governors chose to define the Council's purposes and scope broadly and employed maximum restraint in spelling out its formal structure. There was nothing unique about the architecture of the Council; similar interdepartmental bodies exist in New York and elsewhere.[3] It is noteworthy, however, that New York governors did not elect to manage the performance of the Council by manipulating its basic structural features. For example, they did not try to link the Council more closely to their own office through control of its staffing. Nor did they attempt to shape the rules of the game, for instance by asking for majority and minority reports on controversial issues. There is no implication in these observations that the governors in question behaved unusually; other interdepartmental committees generally have been treated in a similar way. However, the behavior of the chief executives tells us something more about the Council.

One important qualification bears special mention. In organizing the Council, two governors, Dewey and Rockefeller, tended to regard the interests of the Department of Health as primary. Although he did not say so in his directive setting up the Council, Governor Dewey made the Commissioner of Health chairman ex officio, which of course gave the Department of Health a tactical advantage during the IHC period, 1946–1956.[4] Similarly, at the time of the reorganization in 1960, Governor Rockefeller proposed that the mechanism be reconstituted as an advisory committee to the Department of Health under the chairmanship of the Commissioner of Health.[5] However, such an arrangement, which

3. Phillips Bradley, "Interlocking Collaboration in Albany," *Public Administration Rev.*, XVII (Summer 1957), 180–87.

4. See Note 1, Chap. 2, p. 24.

5. *Proposed Reorganization of the Executive Branch of New York State Government, Report to Governor Nelson A. Rockefeller* (Albany, N. Y., Dec. 1959), p. 69.

would have been a step backwards, was successfully opposed by the members, including the Department of Health.

Sources of Agenda Items

Chief executives and others seldom attempted to influence the choice of agenda items. Although the Council was accountable to the governor, and also was reponsible to the legislature during the IHRB phase, 1956–1960, when it was an independent agency, its members initiated almost all of its business. The former executive director estimated that the agencies, including the Council staff, initiated about 90 percent of all agenda items during the IHRB period, 1956–1960. All other sources, including the governor, accounted for the remaining 10 percent. The executive secretary of the IHHC as well as the secretary during the IHC period, 1946–1956, also confirmed that much the same pattern prevailed during their years of service. Although no attempt has been made to classify and tabulate agenda items by source, a careful reading of all of the agenda and minutes since the Council's beginning in 1946, and interviews of many persons who participated in meetings, corroborate the judgment of the staff. If anything, such sources suggest that the proportion of agenda items initiated by the members, including the staff, may even be higher. Furthermore, a similar pattern prevailed in the area of rehabilitation, in which the issues were classified. For example, even though the figures on the initiation of rehabilitation issues substantially overestimate the proportion of agenda items referred by outside sources, 70 percent of all the rehabilitation issues that came before the Council were first initiated by the agencies and the staff (45 of 64).[6]

6. The data on rehabilitation issues tend to overestimate the influence of governors and other outside sources in the selection of agenda items because most of the issues extended over months or years and usually were reflected in many agenda items, the great preponderance of which were brought up by the members. The significance of this situation is all the greater, since governors and other external sources rarely attempted to influence the outcome of Council deliberations or to follow up on the issues that they initiated. The procedures followed in classifying rehabilitation issues are

Of the external sources of agenda items, only three are sufficiently significant to warrant discussion: the governor, including his staff; the legislature; and private interest groups. Private interest groups seem to have made somewhat more requests of the Council than either the governor or the legislature, especially during the IHRB phase, when the mechanism had its greatest visibility and seemed to be most influential.[7] For instance, such groups, including the Governor's Council on Rehabilitation, a citizens advisory committee with a special relationship to the Council, which is discussed later, initiated 17 percent of the rehabilitation issues (11 of 64).[8] In sheer number of items introduced, the governor and his staff come next. To illustrate, governors initiated 9 percent of the rehabilitation issues (6 of 64). However, from the members' point of view, chief executives were the most important outside source of requests because of their power. In later years there also was some increase in the number of matters referred by the governor and his aides, even though ironically the Rockefeller administration was less supportive of the mechanism than previous regimes. But this occurred primarily in the area of rehabilitation, in which the Governor had a strong interest. Last, as an initiator of requests, as measured in numbers, but of second greatest importance because of its power, was the legislature. Only 3 percent of the rehabilitation issues were initiated by the legislature (2 of 64). Such interest as this branch of government showed in referring questions to the Council reached

described in the Appendix. Furthermore, there generally was more outside interest in rehabilitation than in other program sectors, particularly since the advent of the Rockefeller administration.

7. There does not seem to be any evidence that the Council, during the IHRB period, 1956–1960, was in fact any more influential with governors or others, except insofar as its responsibilities for temporary operation of certain research and demonstration projects represented a broadening of its role. However, its status as an independent agency with an executive director made it appear to be more influential than it really was.

8. If the Governor's Council on Rehabilitation is excluded from the computations, the proportion of issues initiated by private interest groups drops to 9 percent (5 of 58), and to 8 percent, if it is excluded only from the numerator (5 of 64).

its height during the IHRB period, when relations between the Council and legislature were closest. Then the executive director had a budget to defend and an agency to maintain.

Handling of Agenda Items

More striking than the failure of governors and others to refer questions to the Council was their disinclination to influence the handling of agenda items. On the whole, Council members enjoyed remarkable freedom, for rarely was the Council subjected to much pressure in reaching favorable decisions. The time that Governor Harriman rejected the Council's recommendation that the "disability freeze" provisions of the Social Security Amendments of 1954 be administered by the Division of Vocational Rehabilitation is one of the few exceptions.[9] Moreover, there is no evidence that a governor ever threatened the members with sanctions to gain compliance with his wishes. Most of the issues that governors referred to the Council either did not involve conflict or were defined in fairly noncontroversial terms, so chief executives had little or no need to exert their authority. In addition, chief executives showed little interest in the Council's handling of matters that the members chose to bring up themselves, except when recommendations were made to the governor's office.

Throughout the entire history of the Council, no governor ever attended a meeting. Nor was it customary for gubernatorial assistants to sit in on or participate in meetings. From the inception of the Council in 1946 through 1965, members of the governor's office and representatives of the Division of the Budget attended only 5 of 157 meetings held.[10] Moreover, until fairly late in Council history, it was not common practice to keep the governor informed of Council deliberations by sending his staff copies of the agenda and minutes.[11] It was not until 1962 that a member

9. See pp. 50–52.

10. The total number of meetings may be off from 1 to 3 meetings because of incomplete records.

11. During the IHRB period, 1956–1960, the Council prepared annual reports to the governor and legislature.

of the governor's staff requested that such a practice be instituted. The Council, however, was not the initiator of this practice. The conclusion is inescapable that governors and their staffs did not bother with most of the techniques that could be used to manage the Council or to keep a watchful eye on it.

The Behavior of External Groups and the Value of the Council

Governors

Notwithstanding the fact that they gave the Council free reign, governors found the mechanism to be of value. They therefore helped to sustain it and keep it alive. However, there were marked differences in the perceptions that state administrations had of the Council, and accordingly in their support for it. The behavior of the official family also diverged at times, with the governor's office moving in one direction and the Division of the Budget in another.

The Dewey administration. The Dewey administration thought highly of the Council. Governor Dewey, who in the words of one of his closest aides "was a very administratively sensitive person," felt that interdepartmental councils or committees were very effective coordinating mechanisms. Thus, he utilized the device "more broadly than any previous chief executive."[12]

In spite of Dewey's high regard for the Council, however, he apparently had fairly modest expectations for it as well. As one of the persons who helped staff Council meetings commented, the mechanism was set up "as a means of exchange, a means by which the departments could work together." As such it was viewed as "a forum." Another respondent felt that the Governor's interest in such committees "started with the realization that half of the commissioners didn't know each other." Moreover, Dewey also regarded interdepartmental committees as an alternative to cabinet meetings, which he was not in the habit of calling regularly. To quote a former top aide of the Governor, they

12. Bradley, p. 185.

were thought of as "small cabinets, ad hoc cabinets." Nevertheless, it was intended that the initiative should lie with the member agencies and that they should interact as they thought appropriate. The Governor did not consider the Council, or similar interdepartmental bodies, an integral part of his armory of techniques for active management of the executive branch. Thus during the first decade, the Council operated in the sunshine of the Governor's good will, though not with his active involvement, as one of a number of such instrumentalities.

The Dewey administration therefore encouraged the growth of the Council. After having given birth to the mechanism in 1946,[13] the Governor was pleased to expand its membership in 1953, which the agencies themselves recommended on the suggestion of the Department of Health. During the Dewey regime, the Division of the Budget also acted favorably, if somewhat reluctantly, on the two modest requests that the Council made for temporary staff to assist two of its committees.[14] Throughout the IHC period, 1946–1956, the Council did not have a budget and staff of its own because it was intended that the members were to provide such staffing as was needed.[15] In the words of an aide of the Governor, it was felt "there should be no occasion for additional staff." Moreover, the administration "didn't want such councils to build up as agencies."

On the other hand, there is no evidence that the Council as it was conceived and operated during its first decade ever was considered by the administration to be a liability. Undoubtedly some individuals in state government had doubts about the value of the Council; however, such views never attained any organized expression. The attitudes of the staff of the Division of the Budget

13. The circumstances leading to establishment of the Council are discussed on pp. 24–27.

14. The Committee on Coordination of School Health Services and the Committee on Rehabilitation.

15. As already mentioned, the secretary of the Joint Hospital Survey and Planning Commission, to which most of the Council agencies belonged, served as part-time secretary of the Council during this period. In this he also was assisted by the staff of the Commission. See pp. 26 and 29.

seem to be the sole exception. But since the Council operated without a budget and permanent staff, and thus was considered a low key operation, the Division did not have strong views about the mechanism.

The Harriman administration. The Harriman administration, except for the staff members of the Division of the Budget, also had a high regard for the Council as an administrative mechanism. As the former executive director said, "Harriman was very proud of the IHRB [the Council]." He also extended his predecessor's use of interdepartmental coordinating councils and committees.[16] Not to be outdone, he substantially increased the state's investment in the Council, when, in 1956, he successfully prevailed upon a hostile legislature to raise the mechanism's status to that of an independent agency and give it limited operating functions. His administration also was supportive of the Council's budget requests, but its assistance was qualified by the critical judgment of the Division of the Budget. Like any other agency the Council did not get all that it asked for.

However, Harriman, like Dewey, also conceived of the Council as a body that the member agencies were to run themselves. He and his top aides did not think of it as an instrumentality that it would be advantageous to manage from the executive level. In spite of the fact that the Council had substantially greater stature during the Harriman regime, the administration did not make greater use of it than its predecessor. Likewise, the Council also seems never to have been a problem to the administration. The attitude of the administration toward the Council is best summed up in the remarks of the Governor's secretary: "I felt it was a good thing, but I was not too aware of its operation. . . . It presented no problems for the Governor and his staff. . . . It never was a source of problems or headaches."

The Harriman administration's interest in the Council derived mainly from its unique need to make a record that would keep it in power rather than from any particular administrative convic-

16. Bradley, pp. 186–87.

tions. Not only was Averell Harriman the first Democrat to sit in the governor's chair in twelve years, but as a member of the Division of the Budget said, the Dewey regime was "a difficult show to follow." Dewey had given New York more than a decade of progressive government and he had acquired a reputation as a good administrator. Moreover, Harriman won in a close election, which he was not expected to win, and not against Dewey himself, who had chosen to retire from public life. He also was confronted with a hostile Republican legislature anxious to embarrass him at every opportunity. Therefore, when the fledgling administration assumed office, it searched for desirable programs. One of its first ventures was an expansion and upgrading of the Council. How it did so is worth relating because it illuminates the value the administration placed on the instrumentality.

Governor Harriman was advised to reorganize the Council by the Commissioner of Health. When being interviewed by the Governor's top advisors shortly before the inauguration, the Commissioner of Health was asked for ideas to help formulate a program for the administration. Seeing an opportunity to draw a number of health functions closer to his Department and reduce the burden of interdepartmental meetings, the Commissioner of Health suggested that the new administration create a new Interdepartmental Council on Human Resources by combining the Council with three other interdepartmental bodies: the Joint Hospital Survey and Planning Commission; the Youth Commission; and the Mental Health Commission.[17] The Governor and his advisors liked the idea. It promised to improve state administration through better coordination of health activities, and there was reasonable expectation that it would. Moreover, the proposal was modest and unlikely to arouse partisan objections.

Most of the other Council members were very unhappy when

17. The Commissioner of Health made a similar recommendation to his colleagues on the Council in 1952, but they rejected it (memorandum from Dr. Hilleboe to Members of Interdepartmental Councils and Commissions, Reorganization of Councils, Commissions, and Committees, Nov. 7, 1952).

they learned of the administration's intentions. They feared that the plan would help the Department of Health expand its functions, by giving the Department a better medium for pursuing its objectives, and through reassignment of some of the operating functions of the interdepartmental bodies to be abolished in the proposed reorganization. The Department of Health particularly hoped to absorb the operating responsibilities of the Joint Hospital Survey and Planning Commission, which administered the federal Hill-Burton funds for construction of hospitals and related facilities, a program which in most states was implemented in the health departments.

The other Council members were, in effect, presented with a *fait accompli* and also were in a poor position to object to an administrative move by the new Governor. The Department of Mental Hygiene also was under the direction of an acting commissioner. Consequently, they assented after a Council discussion of the question in January, 1955, in which the Governor's Secretary participated. In a memorandum to the Governor, which was approved at the next meeting, the agencies recommended that Governor Harriman "create by executive order a new Interdepartmental Council on Human Resources with additional members, and a broadened scope, but solely advisory."[18]

Nevertheless, since the details had yet to be worked out, some of the members used the opportunity to persuade the administration to move slowly and limit the scope of the reorganization. The administration soon began to sense resistance to the proposal, especially to including the Joint Hospital Survey and planning Commission and the Youth Commission in the new Council. After eight months of negotiations and delay, in part resulting from some ambivalence in the administration, a compromise finally was reached by the agencies and the Governor's Secretary at the October, 1955, meeting of the Mental Health Commission, an agency to which each of the core agencies also belonged. It was

18. Memorandum from Dr. Herman E. Hilleboe, Chairman, Interdepartmental Health Council, to Hon. Averell Harriman, Feb. 21, 1955, p. 2.

agreed to combine the Council with the Commission, which was expiring, and to establish the merged body through legislative action, primarily because then it would have a separate budget and staff. The finishing touches were put on the plan a month later at a joint meeting of the Council and the Mental Health Commission, when the recommendations of a committee of deputies that had been appointed to negotiate the remaining details were accepted. The Governor's office did not send a representative to this meeting, as the administration was satisfied to let the agencies make the final arrangements.

On January 17, 1956, a year after the first Council discussion of the subject, Governor Harriman, in a special health message to the legislature, presented the recommendations for reorganization of the Council.[19] Faced with a hostile legislature, he leaned heavily upon the argument that the agencies had suggested the changes ("I concur in these constructive recommendations . . .").[20] For the same reason, the Governor's office also asked a staff member of the Mental Health Commission to handle the lobbying for the bill, which Democratic legislators introduced in the assembly and the senate in February. The Republican leadership promptly tabled it for over six weeks. Finally it was released and passed on April 2, 1955, the last day of the legislative session.[21]

The establishment of the Council as a separate agency with some operating responsibilities, however, opened up fissures in the Governor's staff. Whereas previously the Division of the Budget had not shown "too much interest and too much concern," to use the words of a former aide to the Council, because for one thing, "it didn't cost them anything," the Division was very unsympathetic to the reorganized Council. Indeed, it would have opposed the reorganization, but could not, for, as a member of the Division said, "The item was pretty high on the Harriman agenda." The Division's uncharacteristically terse "approved with-

19. "Message Concerning Public Health and Mental Hygiene, January 17, 1956," *Public Papers of Governor W. Averell Harriman, 1956* (Albany, N. Y., n.d.), p. 49.

20. *Ibid.*

21. See Note 14, Chap. 2, p. 30.

out comment" on the bill to set up the reformed Council was indicative of its lack of enthusiasm. In spite of having a poor opinion of the Council ("much ado about nothing") the staff of the Division respected Governor Harriman's commitment to the Council. Although they reviewed the Council's budget requests rigorously, they acted fairly. Certainly, this was the feeling of the executive director of the Council: "The budget examiner was most sympathetic . . . I never had any reason to believe the budget division was unfavorable." But just as assuredly, the Division was not lavish with resources or praise either, as was most evident after the advent of the Rockefeller era.

The Rockefeller administration. In contrast to their predecessors, Governor Rockefeller and his top aides showed no enthusiasm for the Council. In the form in which they inherited the instrumentality, they regarded it as a liability. In fact, the member agencies and others who were knowledgeable felt that the Governor's aides "would have let the whole thing die," if the members, under the leadership of the Commissioner of Health, hadn't persuaded them to compromise. Furthermore, after "cutting the Council down to size" in the reorganization of 1960, the Rockefeller administration mainly tolerated it, a position which weakened the mechanism and created uncertainty about its future. However, with the passing of years, which have been marked by a prodigious growth of new programs having interdepartmental implications, the administration became more favorably disposed toward the Council.

The Rockefeller administration's low opinion and consequent lack of support of the Council was primarily an expression of the administrative philosophy and style of the Governor's office. Its perceptions of the instrumentality, unlike those of its predecessors, was informed by a thoughtful and well-articulated rationale rooted in the academic and practical discipline of public administration. In fact, the most influential exponent of the administration's views, the Governor's Secretary, was a former dean and professor of public administration. It therefore is important to examine the administration's views and to show how they influenced its regard for the Council.

From the outset, the Rockefeller administration was committed to reorganizing the executive branch of the state in the spirit of the famous Hoover commissions. In his first message, the Governor informed the legislature that he was initiating a study, "with a view toward reorganization to achieve greater efficiency, economy, and improved services."[22] The administrative concepts underlying the effort were in the direct lineage of the major federal reorganization studies and the many offspring that these studies spawned at the state and local level. However, unlike most of its forerunners, the study was undertaken by the Governor's office, under the direction of the Governor's Secretary, rather than by a special commission or outside group.

The reorganization study was based mainly upon the application of three traditional principles of administration aimed at strengthening the Governor's hand as chief executive.[23] These "sound management principles," as disclosed in the final report, were:[24]

1. There should be clear lines of responsibility to the Governor.

> The plan proposes: 1. Substantial reorganization of the present executive structure to provide the Governor with clear lines of authority for directing operations of the Executive Branch.[25]

2. The Governor's span of control should not be excessive.

22. *Message of Governor Nelson A. Rockefeller to the Legislature, January 7, 1959,* Legislative Document No. 1 (Albany, N. Y., 1959), p. 20.

23. Herbert Kaufman interprets the reorganization movement as an expression of the quest for executive leadership: "'Concentration of authority and responsibility,' 'functional integration,' 'direct lines of responsibility,' 'grouping related services,' 'elimination of overlapping and duplication,' and 'need for coordination' echoed through state capitols, city and town halls, and even some county court houses as chief executives became the new center of governmental design." See Herbert Kaufman, "Emerging Conflicts in the Doctrines of Public Administration," *American Political Science Rev.,* L (Dec. 1956), 1057–73.

24. *Proposed Reorganization of the Executive Branch of New York State Government* (Albany, N. Y., 1959), p. 1.

25. *Ibid.,* p. 2.

In 1927 there were 65 agencies reporting to the Governor; today there are 136. The Secretary's report deals with 106 of these. . . . The report recommends that the number of State agencies reporting to the Governor . . . be reduced from 106 to 41.[26]

3. Like or related functions should be grouped organizationally.

There are activities which should be closely related but are now separately, even distantly, administered. These obviously should be under unified policy direction and control.[27]

The Council, therefore, was in jeopardy from the outset of the new administration. First, it stood in the path of one of the prime objectives of the reorganization plan, namely to reduce the number of separate agencies reporting to the Governor. But, as an independent interdepartmental agency, the Council also seemed to violate most of the other canons of management to which the Governor and his top aides subscribed. Primarily they felt that in undertaking "research programs," the Council had "carried on activities that belong [ed] to one or more of the member departments."[28] In the eyes of the administration, the Council "had become an operating agency," as a member of the Governor's office said, and to this it was opposed in principle.[29] In the words of our respondent, "Agencies with statutory responsibility should be accountable. It shouldn't be a committee. The Board [the Council] was a collection of responsibilities belonging to various departments." Apparently, there was no implication that the Council had ineffectively performed its activities. The issue was

26. *Ibid.*
27. *Ibid.*, p. 1.
28. *Ibid.*, p. 69.
29. A number of state officials have pointed out that there always has been a strong bias in state government against interdepartmental bodies having operating functions. They reported that Dewey was opposed to this, and that even the Harriman administration was ambivalent on this point. However, there seems little doubt that the Rockefeller administration has been even more strongly opposed and has defined the term "operating" much more broadly than its forerunners, especially in its early years.

organizational. A person who helped to direct the reorganization study indicated that the Governor's office also "felt the Board [the Council] would become a permanent agency."

The administrative concepts to which the administration subscribed also made it see the need for interdepartmental coordination somewhat differently from its precursors. Governor Rockefeller and his advisors tended to view problems of interagency coordination as matters that can be solved through proper departmental assignment of like or related functions.[30] In seeing such problems as questions of formal organization they were therefore inclined to see little value in the Council, other than as a medium for the members "to exchange information regularly on matters of common interest."[31]

The administration, when it assumed office, also apparently considered the Council something of an obstruction to the power of the Governor. At least that was the impression of some individuals aware of opinions in the upper echelons of the state. The Council "might detract from the Governor's power; it might give the commissioners a chance to gang up on the Governor," as one informant said. But, equally important, the mechanism did not synchronize with the administration's style of operation, which was to centralize decision-making in the Governor's office and to assume greater initiative in policy formulation. This necessarily meant greater reliance on dealing unilaterally and somewhat more at arm's length with state agencies.

Moreover, all other factors being equal, the administration was hardly inclined to look favorably upon an institution that was closely identified with the Governor's predecessor, a Democrat. Consequently, feeling strongly about the Council, the administra-

30. James G. March and Herbert A. Simon indicate that "one peculiar characteristic of the assignment problem, and of all the formulations of the departmentalization problem in classical organization theory, is that, if taken literally, problems of coordination are eliminated." See *Organizations* (New York, 1958), pp. 22–29.

31. *Proposed Reorganization of the Executive Branch,* p. 69.

tion proposed drastic surgery. In the report of the reorganization study, it recommended:

> The research projects of the Interdepartmental Health Resources Board [the Council] should be transferred to appropriate State departments, and the Board reconstituted as an advisory committee attached to the Department of Health.
>
> . . . .
>
> With the Commissioner of Health as Chairman, and with such staff services as are necessary supplied by the Department of Health.[32]

For all practical purposes this would have emasculated the Council and ended its life as an interdepartmental body.

Recognizing the danger and feeling strongly about the value of the mechanism, the Commissioner of Health urged his colleagues to join in asking the administration to reconsider. However, the Commissioner of Social Welfare and particularly the Commissioner of Mental Hygiene apparently preferred to let the mechanism die, as long as the Council's dissolution would not bring undue embarrassment. Nevertheless, they went along, mainly because they did not want to get into a fight with the Commissioner of Health and because the Council helped them to keep an eye on his department. Consequently, they wrote the Governor's Secretary urging continuance of the Council. Some support for the Council also developed in other quarters, even before issuance of the Governor's reorganization plan. In its first report to the Governor, the newly formed Governor's Council on Rehabilitation urged him to "continue this effective and quite unique interdepartmental agency . . . if for no other reason than the continuing need for this interdepartmental approach to the broad field of rehabilitation."[33] In an interview the chairman reported, "We had a conviction that a board [council] or something like it was essential." The Rehabilitation Council already

32. *Ibid.*

33. Report to the Governor from the Governor's Council on Rehabilitation, p. 3. Enclosed with letter from Leonard W. Mayo, Chairman, to The Honorable Nelson A. Rockefeller, Dec. 21, 1959.

had developed "a good relationship" with the Council and also was dependent upon it for staff and easy access to the member departments. In addition, the Joint Legislative Committee on Mental Retardation "expressed its complete support for the Board [the Council] and indicated that it would support any form of continuing legislation that might be introduced.[34] Some support also came from at least one of the major voluntary health agencies concerned with rehabilitation.

The matter finally was compromised late in January, 1960, at a meeting attended by several of the commissioners, the Governor's Secretary, and representatives of the Division of the Budget. The Governor's Secretary agreed to ask the Governor to continue the Council by executive order upon expiration in March, 1960, of the 1956 statute under which the Council had operated for four years.

The Rockefeller administration also failed to support the Council, or gave it slight support, after the reorganization. Perhaps of foremost importance, the administration initiated or agreed with efforts between 1959 and 1962 to establish four citizens' advisory committees, three of which tended to limit the Council's sphere of influence. However, the limitations resulted coincidentally rather than intentionally, and more through oversight than by deliberate design.

Several episodes concerning the four citizens' advisory committees are worth relating. The first occurred even before the reorganization, when the Governor moved to set up a citizens' advisory committee on rehabilitation.[35] Rehabilitation, of course, was the policy sphere in which the Council had been most active. Moreover, the Council was accustomed to having its own citizens' advisory committees in some of the policy areas in which it operated, and had given some thought to creating such a committee in rehabilitation. The agencies felt particularly that a citizens'

34. Minutes of the IHRB, December 22, 1959, p. 2.

35. "Message Recommending a Rehabilitation Program for Disabled Citizens of the State, March 16, 1959," *Public Papers of Governor Nelson A. Rockefeller, 1959* (Albany, N. Y., n.d.), p. 121.

committee with direct access to the Governor might threaten their interests. Unless the committee were closely allied to the Council, the members might be put in a "defensive position" and "never know what was going on." Consequently, they asked the Governor's staff to link the new committee to the Council in two ways: make it advisory to the Council as well as to the Governor, and arrange for the Council to staff it. Both requests were granted. As it turned out, the Governor's Council on Rehabilitation, which the committee was called, was an unintended blessing in disguise. It not only supported the Council, but it was another route by which the members gained gubernatorial support for their rehabilitation programs.

However, the Council did not fare as well in the other policy spheres in which attempts were made following the reorganization to set up citizens' advisory committees (alcoholism, mental retardation, and narcotics addiction), two of which came to fruition (alcoholism and narcotics addiction). Each of the proposed committees was also to operate in policy areas in which the Council was active; moreover, in two of these areas the Council had had its own committees prior to the reorganization. In the area of mental retardation, the Council had decided to reestablish its own committee, a decision about which the administration probably was not aware. Moreover, none of the new proposals provided for ways in which the advisory committees could follow the pattern of the Governor's Council on Rehabilitation. According to a member of the Governor's staff, "There was no intention of following the pattern of the Governor's Council on Rehabilitation." Unwittingly or otherwise, the administration helped to reduce the Council's sphere of influence, for the two committees that were set up were not linked to the Council in any way.[36]

Although the Governor did not follow through after publicly

36. Both the Advisory Council on Alcoholism and the Council on Drug Addiction were made advisory to the Department of Mental Hygiene alone. The former originally was created by executive order on June 16, 1961, and in 1965 was given a statutory basis (Sec. 302, Mental Hygiene Law). The latter was established by statute in 1962 (Sec. 201, Mental Hygiene Law).

announcing his intention, the administration's attempt to set up a citizens' advisory committee on mental retardation particularly undercut the Council and demonstrated that the Governor and his staff could not be counted on to support the Council mechanism. The ensuing events, which are to be understood in the context of efforts of the Department of Mental Hygiene to partially disengage itself from the Council by exploiting the climate of opinion in the administration, are important enough to relate. First, the Council agreed in November, 1961, to reestablish its own advisory committee on mental retardation.[37] The Commissioner of Mental Hygiene then privately suggested that the Governor establish such a committee, in all probability to head off the Council, and two months later he notified the Council members of the Governor's intentions. He asked them to delay further action on setting up a committee of their own, which they, of course, agreed to do. A week later, on January 30, 1962, the Governor, in a special message to the legislature on mental health, announced his plan to appoint a citizens' advisory committee on mental retardation, but in doing so he neither indicated to whom the committee would be responsible or what, if any, relationship it would have to the Council.[38]

This signaled the start of a protracted, behind-the-scenes struggle among the members over the proper relationship of the proposed committee to the Council and to the Department of Mental Hygiene. On one side was the Commissioner of Mental Hygiene, who at first was agreeable to the committee's being advisory to the Council as well as to the Governor and to his own department, provided that both the advisory committee and the Council's subcommittee on mental retardation were staffed by his agency. Aligned against him were the other commissioners (except the Superintendent of Insurance, who took no position), who wanted the committee to be advisory to the Council in the same fashion

37. Minutes of the IHHC, Nov. 28, 1961, pp. 6–7.

38. "Message Presenting a Comprehensive New Master Plan in Aid of the Mentally Disabled, January 30, 1962," *Public Papers of Governor Nelson A. Rockefeller, 1962* (Albany, N. Y., n.d.), p. 37.

as the Governor's Council on Rehabilitation. The issue almost came to a head six months later, at the Council meeting in August, 1962, but the Commissioner of Mental Hygiene prevented a showdown by requesting that the matter "be tabled until a Fall meeting of the Council."[39]

The issue came up again about half a year later, in February, 1963, when the Commissioner of Mental Hygiene "announced that the governor's office planned to appoint an Advisory Committee on Mental Retardation which would be attached to the Department of Mental Hygiene."[40] This was too much for the other members, most of whom had a large stake in mental retardation. The Council therefore agreed to ask the Governor's office to delay action until both sides could be heard. (This was one of the few times that the members did not present a united front to the governor.) However, when presented with the question, the Governor decided not to act. Three departments were aligned against one, and one of the influential private interest groups in the field backed the majority in the Council. Certainly, the outcome showed that there was little support for the Council within the administration.

The Council's requests for funds also fared poorly under the Rockefeller regime. Although the administration lived up to its agreement, made at the time of the reorganization, to staff the mechanism, it steadfastly opposed any growth of the staff. Each year, beginning with 1962, the members asked for modest increases in staff and each year the Division of the Budget disapproved their request. The only exception further underscored the diminished stature of the Council. In 1963, the administration granted a temporary increase of three positions to man a project of the Governor's Council on Rehabilitation, a project of particular interest to the Governor. Even this request was initially disallowed by the Division of the Budget. It was granted only after the Rehabilitation Council appealed to the Governor's office.

39. Minutes of the IHHC, August 7, 1962, p. 7.
40. *Ibid.*, Feb. 26, 1963, p. 5.

The administration, however, eventually relaxed its objection to the Council's performing certain operating functions. In 1962, the Governor's Secretary supported the members when they asked if the Council could receive outside monies, such as federal funds, to conduct studies and projects. However, permission was contingent upon the funds being handled by the member agencies.

Notwithstanding the Rockefeller regime's low opinion of the Council, it nevertheless provided in its administrative lexicon for interdepartmental coordinating committees. A member of the Governor's staff said that he felt it was too strong to say that the administration merely tolerated the Council, although he agreed that it was skeptical, unconvinced about what such committees can accomplish. Committed as they were to reorganization of the executive branch, the Governor and his aides necessarily had to emphasize the virtues of "sound management principles" and minimize their limitations. Milton Musicus, an official who helped direct the reorganization study, pointed this out in an article on governmental reorganization that appeared five years later in a leading professional journal. He wrote:

> Recognizing that the mere mention of reorganization can mobilize a great deal of opposition, the chief executive often presents the need for reorganization to the public at large on the basis of the strongest and the most universally appealing reason—that of bringing about efficiency and economy in government. This helps mobilize massive support which it is hoped will overcome anticipated opposition to specific proposals. In effect, what is labeled as reorganization is presented as a program of management improvement.[41]

In the later years of the Council there also seems to have been a mellowing of tone, if not an increasingly receptive attitude, in the Governor's office concerning the value of the Council. In speaking of the mechanism, a member of the Governor's office said that he could see the difference in the Council departments' "*élan* and knowledge of each other" compared with the relations

41. Milton Musicus, "Reappraising Reorganization," *Public Administration Rev.*, XXIV (June 1964), 108.

among other state agencies. "There is no doubt about the value of this programmed communication." Certainly, the Council was no longer perceived as a threat or impediment to the Governor's direction of the executive branch. A former member of the Governor's staff said: "The Council does not serve the Governor's needs, but it is not in conflict with them either." This statement suggests that considerable philosophic distance was traversed after the Rockefeller administration first set eyes upon the Council. If the Musicus article is an indication, the administration even began to question some of the principles on which it based its original recommendation to abolish the instrumentality:

> Criteria for judging organizations do not apply to large scale governmental operations with the same validity they do to business or small government agencies. Whereas one speaks normally of a span of control of about 5 to 15 subordinates, the chief executive may find that within a large governmental environment, he can direct more than 100 agencies. He has learned that, with his executive powers, personal prestige, influence, persuasion, and the aid of his staff of program and budgetary personnel, he can exercise supervision over many and diverse activities.[42]

The Division of the Budget

Of all the units of the state government that were concerned with the Council, the Division of the Budget was the least enamored of the mechanism. A member of the governor's staff reported that even during the Rockefeller era the governor's office looked more favorably upon the Council than did the Division. However, in the later years, as problems of interdepartmental coordination became more complex with the growth of new programs, some of the staff of the Division began to reconsider the possible value of interdepartmental coordinating committees.

To understand the Division's view of the Council, it is necessary to look at the exigencies that the Division faces in carrying out

42. *Ibid.*, p. 109.

its functions and the way it is inclined to see problems of interdepartmental coordination.

The search for "rational" control of decision-making—in "technical" as contrasted with "political" terms—underlies the Division's position, and its failure to achieve such control is its greatest source of anxiety.[43] Concerned as it is with evaluating and deciding upon the merits of a vast and complex array of demands upon the limited financial resources of the state, the Division constantly is looking for objective criteria by which to define issues and to render defensible judgments. This responsibility has called for heavy reliance upon quantifiable standards that can be translated into dollar-and-cent terms and emphasis upon proper organization and administration. As technical specialists, budget examiners tend, therefore, to be biased in favor of quantifiable measures of agency performance. As a member of the governor's office commented about budget officials, "For them, the more quantifiable a thing, the greater its worth, and vice versa." Budget personnel also are inclined to be wary, if not suspicious, of the political process.[44] Although they may have to consider political factors, they usually do so reluctantly, for to do so compromises their art and weakens their position. After all, others are better placed to make political decisions than they. Moreover, since budgeting is a continuous cyclical process (annual in New

43. In a case study of the budget process in New York, Paul Appleby, Governor Harriman's Budget Director, is quoted as saying, after reflecting on an episode in which political considerations had overshadowed fiscal ones: "We ought, if we can, to devise a tactical approach that better anticipates the course the opposition will take in a particular legislative session. . . . I think that we ought somehow to be firmer masters of the executive position and thereby in greater measure masters of the legislative product, in spite of all difficulties." These remarks take on particular poignancy when one considers that New York has one of the strongest budget divisions in the nation and is a state accustomed to strong executive leadership of the legislature. See Donald G. Herzberg and Paul Tillett, *A Budget for New York State 1956–1957,* The Inter-University Case Series No. 69 (University, Ala., 1962), p. 31.

44. For a good discussion of the political aspects of budgeting, see Aaron B. Wildavsky, *The Politics of the Budgetary Process* (Boston, 1964).

York), budget officials are accustomed to action; and usually they are unable to avoid controversial decisions by stalling.

These exigencies were necessarily reflected in the Division's regard for the Council. The comments of several professionals within the Division clearly illustrated this: "Interdepartmental bodies don't sharpen issues; they compromise everything." There was "too much trade off." The Council was "long on discussion and weak on problems." "It hasn't come to grips with the central problems," such as the realignment of health functions. Furthermore, "The whole process is slow, not pitched to action." Obviously, Division personnel felt that the Council should resolve controversial issues and that it was too political. Budget staff were inclined, rightly or wrongly, to judge the mechanism by criteria that are consonant with their own work.

The strategic exigencies of the Division's position also colored its view of the Council. As a central control agency trying to brake the seemingly insatiable appetite of state agencies for more and more resources, the Division is by necessity acutely alert to strategies and maneuvers to expand agency domains. Consequently, it was concerned about the members' use of the Council to increase pressures for new and expanded programs. For example, this concern, which reached its height during the IHRB period, was clearly manifested by the Deputy Director in a 1957 memorandum to the Governor's Secretary, in which he expressed alarm over several Council recommendations for new programs. He even raised the question of whether it was too late to inform the members of the Council that "its role is to make studies and analyze problems but not necessarily to address themselves to action proposals and recommendations."[45] Obviously, the Division is in a strong position dealing unilaterally with the agencies. Division strategy, according to one of the commissioners, is "to play one department off against another."

At times, the Division also viewed the Council as a competitor

45. Memorandum from Clark Ahlberg, Deputy Director, to Jonathan Bingham, Secretary to the Governor, September 11, 1957.

if not a potential threat to its functions. Several members of the Division who were interviewed voiced objections that some of the functions performed by the staff of the Council "really are budget functions." There was sentiment within the unit, at least after the reorganization of the Council in 1956, for tying the mechanism more closely to the governor's staff, particularly to the Division itself. This obviously would have removed any threatening aspects of the Council and probably would have aided the Division in carrying out its coordinating functions. For example, at the time the Council was made an independent agency, several key staff members preferred to see the mechanism tied to the governor's office and to let the Division "ride herd on the interdepartmental setup." Certainly, all indications suggest that the leaders of the Division would have opposed further strengthening of the Council, unless they were assured adequate control of it. Later indications of a more favorable attitude about the possible value of the Council in part reflected a feeling that the instrumentality might be useful to the Division and the governor's office, if properly managed by them.

The Legislature

The Council was neither an asset nor a liability to the legislature. Legislators rarely had much to do with the mechanism; the Council simply did not perform any important functions for them. In fact it is difficult, if not incorrect, to speak of the legislature as having had an attitude or point of view toward the Council.

On the whole, interdepartmental instrumentalities such as the Council have been regarded by legislators as "executive mechanisms" and thus none of their concern. As a key staff aide of the state senate said, "It has been a traditional rule in the legislature not to interfere with the internal management of the executive branch." This explains why the lawmakers ultimately assented to Governor Harriman's request in 1956 to set up the Council as an independent agency. From their point of view the bill "didn't create anything of substance." The Republican leadership stalled the bill merely to embarrass the Governor and to improve its bargaining position. Consequently, the legislature was not very aware of the Council. A former staff aide to the Joint Legislative Committee on Mental Retardation and Physical Handicap indicated that this obliviousness prevailed even during the IHRB period, when the Council had a budget and program to defend: "I don't think many legislators knew it existed."

The legislature also was not responsive to efforts that would draw it closer to the Council. On the few occasions that the member agencies made overtures to legislators to attend Council meetings, their efforts usually came to naught. For example, a former staff member of the Council reported that in the mid 1950's the assembly majority leader was invited to attend but that he did not come. Furthermore, the committees of the legislature usually preferred to deal with the Council agencies directly rather than go through the Council.

Assemblyman Mailler's membership in the Council between 1946 and 1954 was the only continuing link between the legislature and the Council. Yet, although Mailler was a faithful and interested member (he attended 71 percent of the meetings), his participation was personal rather than institutional. It derived from an interest in interdepartmental coordination that he developed while heading the Mailler Commission, not from his position as majority leader. Thus, when Mailler retired from the legislature in 1954, this link was broken and was not restored.

Private Interest Groups

Second to governors, private interest groups benefited most from the Council. Mainly, it provided them with an additional route by which they occasionally were able to influence the member agencies. However, such value as the Council had for them in this respect was very limited. Since the two centers of power within the state government, the governor and the legislature, did not press the Council to make controversial decisions, private interest groups did not find the mechanism too useful a fulcrum for exerting their influence.

In addition to being able to put limited pressure on the members by referring issues to the Council, private interest groups found the instrumentality helpful by their being represented on Council advisory committees. In this way they were able to make their views better known to the agencies. However, such power as they were able to wield in this way was often more apparent than real. As one of the commissioners said, the Council gave such groups "the feeling that they can meet top people and have some semblance of influence." Furthermore, the value of the Council in this regard was limited to the IHRB period, 1956–1960. The citizens' advisory committees that were formed during that period were not reestablished after the Rockefeller reorganization of 1960.

After its establishment in 1959, the Governor's Council on Rehabilitation was the most important avenue by which private interest groups in the field of rehabilitation influenced the Council. Because of its access to the governor and its unique relationship to the Council, this advisory group gave some influence to the individuals and groups that it coopted. However, in making itself felt, the Rehabilitation Council avoided issues involving fundamental conflict among the Council members. For instance, although it initially received some encouragement from the governor's office to do so, the Rehabilitation Council never took up the question of the division of rehabilitation responsibilities among the agencies. Accordingly, there was a symbiotic quality to the relationship between the two Councils.[46]

46. James D. Thompson and William J. McEwen emphasize that "cooptation affects the co-opted as well as the co-opting party." See "Organizational Goals and Environment," in *Complex Organizations,* ed. Amitai Etzioni (New York, 1961), pp. 177–86.

CHAPTER 7

Differences Among Levels of Coordination

HOW the Council operated at the central and regional committee levels, particularly the latter, was an important aspect of its functioning. In the area of rehabilitation, on which this analysis rests, the regional committees were the only field groups that took root, and they also were the only ones in operation at the time the study was conducted.[1] Furthermore, as has been indicated, rehabilitation is the area in which the Council was most active. Consequently, concentrating upon the mechanism's functioning in this program sector shows the lower levels of operation at their best.

The most striking thing about the subordinate levels of the Council is that the regional rehabilitation committees were of little value, except as a forum.[2] These committees were severely handicapped by the impact on them of the member agencies and the Council. In addition, the goals of the regional committees proved

1. See Note 5, Introduction, p. 4.
2. The similarities in the operation of the central committees and the Council proper were much greater than the differences. Not only did the same informal rules, strategies, and processes prevail at meetings, but the benefits and the costs of participating in the mechanism were much the same at the two levels.

to be unattainable, at least as originally conceived, so there was little for them to do.[3]

The Origins and Development of the Regional Committees

The rehabilitation field committees were born of the Rockefeller administration's search, in its early years, for new and desirable programs that would develop its stature. As a key state official commented, "The Governor was looking for new ideas." Thus, during the administration's study of the Council in 1959, when it was preparing proposals for reorganization of the executive branch, one of the Governor's top aides hit upon the idea of developing a network of state-aided medical rehabilitation centers throughout New York.[4] The plan, which was prepared in the Governor's office in consultation with officials of the Department of Health and other agencies, particularly members of the Committee on Rehabilitation, visualized that:

> The major function of the proposed centers would be to supplement the rehabilitation services rendered by public and private groups in the community and thus provide more effective services to programs administered either directly by the State or by local governments with State aid. [Moreover] State and local governmental agencies would be strongly encouraged to refer their patients or clients to these centers.[5]

Rehabilitation centers are facilities that help handicapped persons, usually the severely disabled, to become as self-sufficient as possible through a wide range of professional services, including

3. In most other respects, the regional committees exhibited essentially the same operating characteristics as the central committees and the Council proper. For instance, they eschewed conflict, observed the same informal rules, and employed the same strategies and processes.

4. For a description of the resulting program by its chief administrator, see Edward R. Schlesinger, "A New Program for the Rehabilitation of the Handicapped," *American J. of Public Health,* LIII (March 1963), 398–402.

5. New York State Organization Study of State Rehabilitation Services, Office of Secretary to the Governor, Oct. 1960, p. 4.

medical, psychological, social, and vocational. Although rehabilitation centers differ according to the types and severity of the conditions of their patients, their approach is typically patient-centered, comprehensive, and interdisciplinary. Such centers also vary in the comprehensiveness of their services, the kinds of services in which they specialize, such as medical or vocational, and whether they have inpatients, outpatients, or both. Moreover, some are independent facilities; some may be divisions of other institutions, such as hospitals, or may be affiliated with them.[6]

The purpose of the new state program was to strengthen a selected number of exisiting hospital-based centers and to stimulate the development of new ones in hospitals that lacked rehabilitation services. Essentially, the centers chosen were to be helped to expand their services and make them more comprehensive through annual operating grants (of up to $50,000) that would make up deficits in operating budgets. The plan specified that the Department of Health would administer the new program and that the Council would coordinate with it the existing rehabilitation programs of the various state agencies. To assist the Council in this task, it was decided that regional rehabilitation committees would be established under the aegis of the Council to coordinate both public and private rehabilitation services at the local level in conjunction with the rehabilitation centers.

Initially, the Governor's office had decided to support two centers on a pilot basis in order to assess the effectiveness of the program, which has come to be known as the Rehabilitation Center Program. However, the public response of private health groups to the Governor's announcement, in October 1960, of the first pilot center in Syracuse was so favorable that the administration quickly moved ahead to implement the full program.[7] An official of the Department of Health commented, "It was the first time we were pushed to do something we wanted to do."

6. For a survey of the dimensions of rehabilitation centers, see Basil J. F. Mott, *Financing and Operating Rehabilitation Centers* (Chicago, 1960).

7. Press Release of Governor Nelson A. Rockefeller, Oct. 17, 1960, Albany, N. Y.

Consequently, it fell to the Council, particularly to the Committee on Rehabilitation, to develop the regional committees. Thus, over a three-year period, 1961 through 1963, the Council set up committees in each of the five regions of the Department of Health outside of New York City, concurrent with the designation by the Department of a "primary" rehabilitation center in each region.[8] (A regional committee was not organized in New York City until 1964, but since it varies structurally in several important respects from the others, it is excluded from this analysis.)[9] As each committee was organized, the heads of the agencies participating in the Committee on Rehabilitation, except for the Insurance Department, assigned a field man to represent his agency.[10] And once they were activated, the regional committees began to meet approximately once each month, except during the summer.

The development of the regional committees was difficult, however, for the original plan was very vague about how the committees were to operate and what functions they were to perform. More significantly, the original plan assumed that the committees and the centers would share a wide range of common interests, an assumption that the subsequent evolution of the committees belied. Although it was ambiguous, the plan anticipated that the regional committees would assist the primary centers to

8. Originally, the Rehabilitation Center Program distinguished between primary, secondary, and other rehabilitation centers, and it called for one primary center and one or more secondary and other centers in each region. However, with the passage of time this distinction increasingly was played down because of the onus that many of the facilities felt is attached to being designated as a secondary center. The original concept that the primary centers would provide more comprehensive services than the other centers and that they would be a hub in and out of which referrals of the most difficult cases would flow to and from the other centers also was borne out in practice to only a limited extent.

9. The New York City committee included representatives of both city and state agencies, had a full-time staff, and was staffed by an office attached to the New York City Department of Health for housekeeping purposes.

10. Although the Division of Parole did not become a member of the Committee on Rehabilitation after the reorganization of 1960 until the spring of 1963, it also was invited to name representatives, which it did.

become "a focus of coordination of medical rehabilitation services," within the areas they served, as well as to induce the referral of patients from government agencies.[11] The close relationship expected between the state agencies represented on the committees and the rehabilitation centers also was reflected in an unusual arrangement that required each primary center to hire a "regional rehabilitation coordinator." This person was given the dual role of (1) assisting the primary and other centers in his region in their external relationships, and (2) of fostering coordination of rehabilitation services among official and voluntary agencies in the region. In the first capacity the regional coordinator was to work under the supervision of the director of the primary center, and in the second, under the direction of the regional committee, of which he also was made the executive secretary.[12]

Consequently, there was considerable confusion, especially during the first few years, as to how the regional committees would assist the centers and how the regional coordinators were to function. On the one hand, the directors of centers were inclined to feel that the regional committees and the regional coordinators were responsible for helping them develop their facilities, and particularly to see that state and local government agencies utilized the centers. On the other hand, the agencies represented on the field committees tended to feel that they had no obligation to assist the centers beyond referring patients to them or encouraging other government agencies to do so when more appropriate facilities were not available. Instead, these agencies preferred to rely on the local rehabilitation services and facilities that in the judgment of their field staffs were better suited to serve them and their clienteles. Granting the centers

11. New York State Organization Study of State Rehabilitation Services, p. 5.

12. Although this arrangement for staffing the regional committees was chosen mainly to avoid the delays and difficulties that setting up a state civil service position would have entailed, it was felt that the dual roles were compatible.

limited financial support, $50,000 per annum in the case of the primary centers, and designating them as part of a network of facilities did not change their services enough to alter appreciably their relations with the state agencies.[13] Moreover, many of the agencies represented on the regional committees, such as the Department of Correction and the Division of Parole, because of the nature of their programs, had little or no occasion to use the rehabilitation centers. Then, too, the field representatives were reluctant to become advocates of the centers, for, in addition to the fact that have had little or nothing to gain from becoming so, such involvement might embroil them in local politics and antagonize competing groups and staffs of other facilities with whom they must get along.

The regional committees, therefore, gradually became disengaged from the rehabilitation centers and instead become government interagency mechanisms serving the rehabilitation interests of the member departments. Although many efforts were made to reconcile the interests of the regional committees and the rehabilitation centers, they were of little avail. For example, the Committee on Rehabilitation several times issued guidelines on the roles of the regional committees and the regional coordinators. The parent committee and its representatives also met with the directors of the rehabilitation centers, the regional coordinators, the chairmen of the regional committees, and the committees themselves. The regional coordinators, who were caught in the middle of diverging interests, even began to meet informally on a fairly regular basis to consider their problems. Yet notwithstanding these and other efforts, the divergence of interests between the committees and the centers increasingly became

13. Although the data available on the number of patients served by the primary centers in the five regions are unreliable (because of inconsistencies in reporting and changes in the definition of the reporting categories), they suggest that the rate of growth of state-sponsored patients has not kept pace with the growth of other patients. (During the first three years of the state program in each of the five primary centers taken as a group, the number of state-sponsored patients grew by 18 percent [206/1141] compared with 27 percent [454/1655] for all other patients.)

apparent and even accepted. Thus, in 1965, four years after the creation of the first regional committee, the parent committee reached the conclusion that

> the full potential of the regional committees . . . [can] not be developed with a part-time regional coordinator who has conflicting allegiance to [the] primary center and [the] regional committee, since this conflict confuses the coordinator himself, his committee and the public image of the function of the committee. The lack of his own secretarial staff . . . [and dependence] upon the needs of the primary center also has worked against a consistent and active program.[14]

Consequently, the Council later attempted to make the regional coordinators full-time state employees solely responsible to the regional committees.

The Committee on Rehabilitation also acted to protect the autonomy of the regional committees from other outside influences, for it rejected the intention of the original plan that the regional committees be composed of both public and private agencies. The Committee's guidelines stipulated that private agencies could be invited to serve only in an advisory capacity on subcommittees, which assured state agency control of the committees and of their relations with the community. In fact, as its minutes reveal, the parent committee even cautioned the regional committees against becoming too involved in community affairs:

> The same discretion should be used [by the regional committees] in facing community issues . . . as would be if the matter were of concern to an individual department. In most instances the committees should avoid aligning themselves on one side or the other when controversial community issues arise.[15]

The evolution of the regional rehabilitation committees became a difficult search for meaningful functions for the committees that

14. Minutes of the Committee on Rehabilitation, Subcommittee on Regional Coordination, IHHC, May 12, 1965, p. 1.

15. Minutes of the Committee on Rehabilitation, IHHC, Oct. 15, 1963, p. 4.

well illustrates the need of organizations to protect their autonomy and to avoid involvements that do not serve their interests.

The Advantages and Disadvantages of the Regional Committees

Although much doubt persisted among their members about the role and future of the regional rehabilitation committees—"We still don't know where we are going"—the committees settled into a fairly stable pattern of behavior. Consequently, a reasonably clear picture of the advantages and disadvantages of participating in the committees emerged. As one of the regional coordinators said of his committee, "We now are at a point after three years where we can see value in it."

The most striking fact about the regional committees is that field personnel found their committees to be less valuable and less threatening than their counterparts on the parent rehabilitation committee. The regional committees also performed somewhat different functions for each group. It is important therefore to look at the benefits and costs of the regional committees from the points of view of agency representatives at both levels.

Benefits and Costs to the Field Representatives

The regional committees primarily served a "useful educational function and opened up informal lines of communication" among the agencies' field offices, to use the words of one of the more sanguine field representatives. Almost without exception the regional committee members who were interviewed (approximately two-thirds of the total members) cited getting to know each other and one another's programs as the most valuable contribution of the regional committees: "The value of the committee is getting to know each other and each other's problems." "To me knowing what the other fellow is doing has been the most fruitful thing, and for him to know my headaches." Yet, although many persons felt that this was a "very productive," "really worthwhile" function, most were hard pressed to give tangible examples of benefits that resulted from it. And most were frank to say that there had been "little carry-over" into their units' operations. Besides creating a better climate among the agencies' field offices and broadening their understanding of rehabilitation, the advantages of the committee interchange were limited principally to occasional facilitation of the referral of patients among the agencies. For example, one committee member reported, "The biggest help is I have gotten to know people in other agencies and learn how to refer problems." Another said, "The committee helped us adapt our rules to working with the other agencies." Still another indicated, "Sometimes there have been discussions of particular patients and a hashing out of a solution; much red tape has been cut through." Nonetheless, results such as these were rare, and usually problems were worked out by the interested parties outside of the committees. The regional committees did not examine and recommend changes in the policies and procedures of the agencies either to the parent committee or to the individual agencies.

The regional committees also helped the agencies' field offices to gain greater knowledge of their localities. They assisted the field representatives mostly through increasing their knowledge of rehabilitation resources in their communities and by fostering understanding of their programs, which probably facilitated referrals to and from the programs and slightly enhanced their agencies' reputations. Consequently, the regional committees were engaged in such activities as visiting rehabilitation facilities in their regions; sponsoring rehabilitation film series and educational meetings that demonstrated their programs; and keeping abreast of local developments relating to rehabilitation by inviting representatives of private and other public agencies as program speakers. On occasion, the regional committees also made recommendations to the parent body about the need for additional rehabilitation facilities in their regions, but the Committee on Rehabilitation was not very responsive to such suggestions. Some of the committees even tried to add a few representatives of private agencies to their membership, but were turned down by the parent committee. Yet, notwithstanding these efforts, the impact of the regional committees in their communities was slight. One committee member admitted that it had taken his committee a long time to make its existence known. Another avowed that he did not think his committee had gotten off the ground in its relations with the community. And one of the regional coordinators even asserted, "Our involvement with the community has been nothing."

Just as field personnel did not find participation in the Council as advantageous as their counterparts at higher levels, they also did not find it as disadvantageous, in the sense of its being threatening to their interests. Although some were apprehensive at the first few meetings of the regional committees, and occasionally "There have been cross currents of controversy below the surface," the deliberations of the regional committees were singularly devoid of conflict. As one of the regional coordinators said, "That kind of question doesn't come up."

The principal costs of involvement were the small return from the time and effort put into the committees and the frustrations resulting from the confusion over their purposes. To illustrate with some representative comments by committee members: "You don't feel it is a terribly important committee; you don't feel any sense of accomplishment." "The meetings take a day out of the life of every member of the committee, to what purpose I'm not sure, and keep him from doing other things." Although many members were hopeful and desirous that their committees would become more useful, considerable frustration arose from the continued uncertainty about the committees' role. Moreover, much of the annoyance was blamed on the Committee on Rehabilitation. Sentiments such as these were common: "We don't know what is expected of our committee." "We are not clear on our relation to the state unit [parent committee]." "We still could get more direction from the parent committee; it would have helped a lot if they had defined our role in the beginning." The regional committees increasingly felt that they needed more staff assistance and a modest budget if they were to accomplish much. That such wishes were not fulfilled, although the

Council latterly took steps to try to satisfy them, added to the committees' frustrations.[16] In fact, there is good reason to doubt that the committees would have survived if the decision had been left to their members. One member said about his committee, "I get the impression it's a meeting we go to because we are supposed to."

The limited value of the regional committees for field personnel was reflected in a lack of interest among the representatives of the four core agencies—Health, Mental Hygiene, Social Welfare, and Education—in leading the regional committees. Contrary to their performance elsewhere in the Council, the core agencies did not attend meetings more frequently than the noncore departments (78 compared with 79 percent), although there was some variation in performance between the two groups among the committees, ranging up to 8 percent. By comparison, the core departments were represented at 97 percent of meetings of the Committee on Rehabilitation, during the IHHC period, whereas the other agencies attended only 72 percent of the meetings of the parent body. Similarly, the core agencies did not dominate the chairmanship of the regional committees. One of the regional coordinators suggested that the core agencies probably had less need for the regional committees than the others, in spite of their greater stake in rehabilitation, because they had working relationships with each other at the field level. None of the agencies, in fact, showed much interest in leading the regional committees. As another regional coordinator said of his group, "They were not dying to be chairmen." Thus the practice of annually rotating the chairmanship among the agencies did not take root at the field level as it did in the Committee on Rehabili-

16. During the latter part of its existence, the Council asked for a modest amount of funds to satisfy these requests in part, and on a trial basis also sought approval to include one of the regional coordinator positions in its budget so that all of the coordinator's time would be devoted to Council business (his regional committee) rather than having to share it with the primary center in his region, as was the case. However, both of these requests were disapproved by the administration.

tation. In many instances, a willing agency representative held the reins for several years.

Benefits and Costs to the Parent Committee

The Committee on Rehabilitation valued the regional committees more than their own members did, partly because it looked upon the committees as extensions of itself. Although it did not conceive the field groups, it was midwife and nurse to them. And, of course, the parent committee was also responsible for carrying out the plan of the governor's office that gave birth to the committees. Consequently, the parent committee necessarily developed a vested interest in their success, for failure of the regional committees certainly would have reflected upon it. However, the Committee's estimate of the regional committees also derived from the functions they performed in its behalf.

The regional committees helped the members of the parent committee somewhat in dealing with their external environment through mitigating outside pressures and in enhancing their agencies' prestige and influence. Of first importance, the regional committees were asked by the Committee on Rehabilitation to serve as advisory groups in the development of two state programs of financial support to local rehabilitation facilities in which it had an advisory role: the Rehabilitation Center Program, which gave birth to the regional committees, and the Sheltered Workshop Support Program, which was administered by the Division of Vocation Rehabilitation of the Education Department. For example, the regional committees were asked to advise on the selection of facilities in their regions to receive state aid under these programs. Accordingly, their members made site visits to facilities, provided background information on applicants, and gave their views of the need of prospective grantees for state assistance. These activities mainly helped to protect those who administered the grant programs from the pressures of applicants seeking to influence decisions, especially from established private agencies. One of the members of the Committee on Rehabilitation reported that the Council had been "used as a front" in the administration of these programs. The regional committees were also called upon occasionally to assist the parent committee in conducting various studies of rehabilitation needs and resources. Moreover, they somewhat enhanced the Council agencies' reputation and influence, not only in activities through their own initiative, but also by helping the Committee on Rehabilitation to sponsor and conduct such educational activities as local conferences for professional and lay leaders.

By contrast, the Committee on Rehabilitation made little use of the regional committees in managing the direct relationships among their programs, for rarely did it request the field groups to consider such relationships. For example, it did not encourage them to consider the adequacy of the policies and procedures for the referral of patients from one agency to another.

As to the disadvantages, the members of the parent body did not find the regional committees to be very threatening. However, they felt them to be more of a potential danger to their agencies' interests than the field representatives. Their concern was evident in various ways. As has been indicated, one of the first things that the Committee on Rehabilitation acted upon when organizing the regional committees was to limit their membership to state agencies, and in fact to the very agencies it represented, even though the original plan suggested that the committees include private as well as public agencies. Then later the Committee rejected the requests of several regional committees to add additional agencies. The parent committee also cautioned the field committees not to get involved in controversial community affairs. Its members were reluctant to go very far in involving the regional committees in the administration of the aforementioned programs of state aid to rehabilitation facilities, for example in helping to choose the facilities to receive state funds. One of the field representatives of an agency administering one of these programs reported that even though he thought it wise to have his committee check up on the facilities receiving departmental funds—because "it would take the pressure off me"—the head of the program "didn't go for it," because "he felt this was a departmental prerogative." The failure of the Committee on Rehabilitation to encourage the regional groups to consider questions involving the agencies' policies and procedures also reflected its members' concern about the autonomy of their programs. Finally, it is evident that the evolution of the regional committees was a frustrating experience for the parent committee. Nonetheless, the Committee on Rehabilitation did not find the regional committees to be very costly, for the field groups were constrained both by their subordinate position and their inherent tendency to avoid embarrassing their members.

Factors that Accounted for the Differences Between the Regional and the Central Committees

Why did the regional committees perform such limited functions and why did the field and central office personnel tend to value them differently? The answer is to be found mainly in the influence of organizational factors inherent in the situation; also the impact of these factors was magnified by certain historical circumstances.

The Level of Hierarchy

The need and possibilities of coordination. Field personnel feel less need for coordinating mechanisms such as the Council than do those at higher organizational levels, for at their rung on the hierarchical ladder (in their agencies) they neither find the external environment as threatening nor the rewards of working out cooperative arrangements among their programs as great. Although field staffs are concerned with outside relations, most of the political and other pressures to which their departments are subjected are focused at the top levels, where the power of decision lies. Maintaining and enhancing the organization is primarily the job of top officials. This helps to explain why the Committee on Rehabilitation was more cautious about the field committees becoming involved with other groups than the committees themselves. An experienced observer of the regional committees noted,

"The state people want contact with voluntary agencies, but they are afraid of it . . . the greatest concern is at the top." Field representatives also are less fearful of each other because their discretion and power are severely limited. There is less meaningful interaction among them. Consequently, they have much less need to keep an eye on each other and test one another's intentions. As one of the regional committee members remarked, "Interdepartmental struggles are at a high level." This comment sheds light on why the Committee on Rehabilitation did not encourage the regional committees to examine the relationships between the policies and procedures of the member agencies. It was too threatening.

Field staff members not only feel less need to coordinate, but they are less able to do so, for their power of decision is tightly circumscribed by the policies and procedures of their departments. Moreover, because of their location at the bottom of the chain of command, they usually have more superiors whom they must consider and watch for cues. Paradoxically, although field representatives often are more attuned to the needs of their agencies' clientele—"We are client-oriented," as one of them phrased it—they are unable to make the changes in the policies and procedures to integrate their agencies' services. The head of a community planning agency who observed the regional committees said, "They can't influence policy very much." This reality was well recognized by most committee members, as some representative comments illustrate: "The committee has no authority." "It is not a policy-making body." "It is hard for a committee like this to accomplish much, since the authority to act rests elsewhere." This fundamental limitation underlay most of the frustration that the members of the regional committees experienced in trying to activate their committees and it helps to explain why the members derived so little from them.

Varying interest in rehabilitation. Another reason why the field representatives did not find the regional committees as useful as did the members of the Committee on Rehabilitation was, surprisingly, that they were less interested in rehabilitation than their superiors in the parent group. This, too, resulted from hierarchical differences. On the whole, the Council agencies assigned the heads of their rehabilitation programs to the central committee and the heads of their field offices, or of major units within them, to the regional committees. Consequently, many of the field representatives had responsibilities for a broader range of departmental programs than the members of the parent body, which diluted their interest in rehabilitation. The effect was counteracted somewhat when top field representatives asked subordinates who were rehabilitation specialists to attend meetings for them. However, such subalterns were even more handicapped in acting for their agencies because of their low status.

Hierarchical distance. The organizational distance between the members of the field committees and the central committee, which inhibited communication between the Council participants within each agency, also handicapped the development of the regional committees and contributed to differing views of them. For example, in no department was the member of the Committee on Rehabilitation the immediate superior of his agency's field representatives. In most instances, the field and the central agency representatives were separated by several organizational layers, and in many were not even in the direct line of command. As a result there was little or no communication between agency representatives regarding Council business. Most communication was conducted by way of the parent committee itself, and this was limited largely to contact between the Council staff and the regional coordinators.

Committee turnover. Because there is more movement at the bottom rungs of the career ladder in an organization than at the top (upward, lateral, and in and out of the organization), the regional committees had to contend with much greater turnover in their membership than the parent committee. One third of the members of the regional committees, taken as a group, made a change at least once in the first three years after each committee was activated. In some committees, more than half of the members were new. Actually, these figures understate the turnover, since they do not take into account the alternates that were asked by the regular members to fill in for them at meetings. By comparison, the membership of the Committee on Rehabilitation changed little from 1960 through 1965, and most agency representatives had long tenures, some since the founding of the committee in 1953.

The turnover in the regional committees made it more difficult for the field groups to accomplish much, for new members needed time for orientation in their own agencies and in the committee. Yet, paradoxically, the changes in the field representatives also helped to sustain interest in the committees, for new members often learned the most from meetings and generated the most interest. The committees helped them to make contacts and to know their way around. As one of the new members said of his participation, "For me it's been particularly helpful."

Differences in agency organization. Differences in the organizational structure of the Council agencies also constituted more of an impediment to operation of the regional committees than to the parent group. Most important, the territories covered by the agencies' field offices varied greatly and generally were not even coterminous with the areas covered by the regional committees. "Our territories are entirely different," was a frequent complaint of committee members. This not only restricted the overlap of agency interests at the field level, but it sometimes created a touchy situation between field offices of the same agency when the geographic area covered by a regional committee encompassed part of the territory of several offices. As one of the committee members said of another who represented his agency in such a situation, "He was never sure how far he could represent his agency."

Because of the differences in the organization of the agencies' field offices, there were also wide variations in the responsibilities and status of the field representatives. For example, the Department of Mental Hygiene was usually represented on the regional committees by heads of state mental hospitals, whereas the Workmen's Compensation Board was usually represented by technicians who processed individual cases. In addition, the accompanying differences in civil service grade impeded joint action, for as one of the regional coordinators observed, "In government, grade implies power and authority." To add to these difficulties, there was great variation among the agencies in the lines of responsibility between the field and central committee representatives.

The Structure of the Council

The development and operation of the regional committees were profoundly influenced by the basic characteristics of the Council. Of greatest importance, the regional committees had to struggle with considerable uncertainty and confusion because the Committee on Rehabilitation was severely handicapped in playing a hierarchical role. Being responsible to the Committee on Rehabilitation, the regional committees expected the parent body to make decisions, particularly to give them direction. Yet, because the parent body lacked authority over the agencies it represented, and thus could act only by unanimous consent, it usually disappointed the wishes of the regional committes for guidance. The frustrations that this engendered were among the field representatives' most frequently expressed annoyances, as the following comments illustrate: "We don't know what is expected of the committee." "The committee doesn't have a clear mandate; the original guidelines read like the preamble to the constitution, and the more recent instructions . . . read like the constitution." "Most of our jobs are pretty well structured; when you get into something like this that is so unstructured, it is difficult." Yet, from its point of view there was not much more that the parent committee could have done to solve the problem other than to move cautiously. Least of all could the committee be expected to admit its inability to act decisively.

The dilemma that the regional committees and the parent group faced in their relations also was reflected in another frequent complaint of the field representatives, namely that they seldom heard from the parent committee on the outcome of their recommendations and that communication was in one direction only—upwards. As one committee member said, "I don't know whether our recommendations are dropping dead or the Committee on Rehabilitation doesn't know how to handle them." Although the Council was clearly handicapped by insufficient staff, the source of much of the silence seems to have been that the parent committee did not know what to say because it could not act on the recommendations.

The members of the regional committees and the parent body were also plagued with an understandable confusion of roles, which produced misunderstandings and disappointments. Because they were members of agencies in which hierarchical authority plays a major part in governing their behavior, sometimes they failed to recognize that the Council called for a different style of behavior between levels as well as within their committees. Consequently, they expected hierarchical behavior from others when it was not possible and they sometimes acted hierarchically when it was inappropriate. This problem was present in the regional committees' expectation of clear decisions from the Committee on Rehabilitation. But it was also evident in the failure of the parent body to appreciate the nature of its relationship to the regional committees. For instance, the parent committee on the one hand encouraged the regional groups to play a significant role and on the other held them back, a duality of attitude that made the regional groups feel all the more frustrated and impotent. "Slapped down" was the expression most frequently used by their members. Another example was a tendency of the members of the parent group to talk down to the regional committees in face-to-face encounters. In one instance, when the Committee on Rehabilitation was the guest of one of the field committees, the members of the parent committee were patronizing to the field group and considered its recommendations in the manner of a hearing board.

Consequently, given the lack of a clear and realizable task for the regional committees, and the impact of the organizational factors that influenced their operation, the development of the committees was necessarily frustrating and their efforts relatively unproductive. Moreover, it was not possible for the Committee on Rehabilitation to give the committees much to do in place of such vague functions as assisting the state-aided rehabilitation centers and trying to coordinate local rehabilitation services, for no member could impose his preferences on another, and each had to feel his way in terms of the possible effect of the committees' behavior on his agency. Something more specific and close to home, such as examining the interrelationships among the agencies' program policies and procedures regarding eligibility and referral of patients would have been too threatening. For the same reason, it also is doubtful that the agencies could have worked out a clear plan of how the regional committees should function prior to setting them up, unless there had been strong gubernatorial pressure to do so. Furthermore, there were no useful precedents. Even if the regional committees had been given a more meaningful and manageable task, they still would have been less productive than either the central committees and the Council proper because of the impact, at their level, of the organizational characteristics of the Council and of the member agencies. Therefore, it is little wonder that one of the commissioners remarked, "I don't think we have gotten the regional apparatus off the ground."

Part III

EVALUATION AND CONCLUSIONS

CHAPTER 8

The Effectiveness of the Council

THE Council was an ineffective instrumentality for making decisions. Not only did it focus its attention upon a limited range of relationships among the member agencies, namely upon the problems of serving such special groups as the physically handicapped and the mentally retarded, but most of its decisions only skimmed the surface of the issues involved. Moreover, few actions or programs undertaken as a result of its decisions probably would not have been undertaken elsewhere or would have been developed much differently had the Council not acted. As a decision-making body, the Council did little more than to make it easier for members to reach agreements and to increase somewhat the likelihood that the objectives agreed upon would be achieved. The Council was, however, rather effective as an instrument of interdepartmental communication.[1]

An Approach to Evaluating the Effectiveness of the Council

The most defensible way of measuring the effectiveness of a formal organization is to consider how well it achieves its an-

1. While providing these benefits, the Council performed for its members the informal functions described in Chap. 3, such as mitigating outside pressures and affording them greater opportunity to observe each other.

nounced goals, for it is in such terms that it justifies its existence and its claims for support.[2] Certainly the governor and the member agencies of the Council would have been pressed to defend the Council against attack if its only purpose had been to serve the maintenance and enhancement needs of its members. An organization does not exist for its own sake alone, least of all a government organization.[3] Thus it is appropriate to consider how well the Council fulfilled the purposes for which it avowedly was established and reorganized several times. In doing so, it also is necessary to take into account major unanticipated consequences, for they may be as significant as intended effects.[4] Finally, in interpreting the results of the Council, it is important to consider how the mechanism's inherent organizational characteristics affected its performance. Failure to do so has led some to underrate and others to overrate the mechanism.

A common problem in implementing the goal attainment approach is to define with sufficient precision, the goals of the

2. Peter M. Blau and W. Richard Scott's definition of formal organizations is relied upon in this discussion. They use the criterion of formal establishment for explicit purposes to distinguish formal organizations from other social organizations. See *Formal Organizations* (San Francisco, 1962), pp. 2–5.

3. Alvin W. Gouldner argues that two distinct models of organization have emerged in the study of formal organizations: a rational model, in which "the organization is conceived as an 'instrument'—that is, as a rationally conceived means to the realization of expressly announced group goals," and a natural system model, in which "the realization of the goals of the system as a whole is but one of several important needs to which the organization is oriented." It is Gouldner's thesis that "one of the central problems in organizational analysis is to reconcile the divergent implications of these two models and to synthesize a new and more powerful model." See "Organizational Analysis," in *Sociology Today,* ed. Robert K. Merton et al. (New York, 1959), pp. 400–27.

4. In a pioneering study of the effectiveness of a program, Herbert H. Hyman and his associates distinguished between four types of effects of a program: intended, unanticipated but desirable, unanticipated undesirable, and anticipated but unintended. This is, however, too refined a classification for our purposes, particularly because of the vagueness of the Council goals. See Herbert H. Hyman, Charles R. Wright, and Terrence K. Hopkins, *Applications of Methods of Evaluation* (Berkeley, 1962), pp. 12–13.

instrumentality to be evaluated, so that they may be used as yardsticks. This difficulty is all the greater with respect to the Council because of the unusual vagueness of its purposes. For example, official documents typically express the Council's goals in such generalities as:

> means for assuring cooperation and interchange of plans within the State administration. . . .[5]
>
> joint and mutual planning and action by several state departments . . . in regard to health and mental health problems of the people of the state which are of direct concern to more than one of the departments of state government. . . .[6]
>
> a vehicle for the continued exchange of information and for cooperative study and action by the State agencies with responsibilities in the fields of health and hospital care. . . .[7]

The customary procedure for meeting the problem of analyzing ambiguous objectives is to measure their achievement indirectly "by translating them into a series of measureable, component, or subsidiary objectives which in totality combine to represent the larger goals."[8] This conceptual step requires interpreting the goals of the organization in the light of both written and oral expressions of them.[9]

Unfortunately it is not possible to translate the Council's goals into very specific objectives without imputing to the mechanism a specificity of purpose it did not possess, for definitive charges played a relatively small part in guiding the behavior of the

5. "Statement–Appointment of Interdepartmental Health Council, October 5, 1946," *Public Papers of Governor Thomas E. Dewey, 1946* (Albany, N. Y., n.d.), pp. 614–15.

6. *New York Laws of 1956,* Chap. 191, Secs. 1 and 3.

7. "Executive Order Establishing an Interdepartmental Health and Hospital Council, March 31, 1960," *Public Papers of Governor Nelson A. Rockefeller, March 31, 1960* (Albany, N. Y., n.d.), pp. 985–86.

8. Hyman, Wright, and Hopkins, p. 5.

9. *Ibid.*, pp. 5–12.

member agencies and others.[10] Views of the Council's objectives that are held by those most familiar with it derive principally from their experience with the instrumentality and the attitudes they brought to it. There was no general agreement among state officials as to what the Council was supposed to do. In addition, the mechanism did not have a clientele to whom it had to justify itself in the vocabulary of explicit purposes, unless its own members and the governor may be considered to have been its clientele. However, the vagueness of the Council's stated goals had advantages, insuring the member agencies' maximum freedom of movement and sparing them and the governor embarrassment from failures to achieve unrealistic expectations.

Difficulty in assessing the effectiveness of the Council is compounded because the results of Council activity are particularly hard to ascertain; their impact was felt largely upon and through other organizations. This difficulty occurs at two levels: the first involving the instrumentality's effect on the activities of the organizations and groups it influenced, principally the member agencies; and the second involving the consequences, attributable to the Council, that these activities had for persons served by the state's health programs. The impact that the Council had upon the state's programs and their clienteles was inextricably tied to the influence of other factors, for the outcome of issues considered by the Council was shaped more by the independent actions of the member agencies, the governor, and others than as a direct result of Council action. Furthermore, the output of the Council derived as much from the exchange of information as from formal agreements.

The foregoing problems constitute formidable, if not insurmountable, obstacles to a rigorous evaluation of the Council's effectiveness. Nevertheless, it is possible to make reasonable judgments about how well the mechanism achieved its purposes and

10. The responsibilities that the Council had during the IHRB period, 1956–1960, for certain research and demonstration projects constituted the sole exception.

what effects it had.[11] The ensuing analysis is limited primarily to the mechanism's impact upon the state's health programs, which were administered principally by the member agencies. It also focuses mainly upon the Council's performance in the area of rehabilitation, the program sector in which the mechanism was generally regarded as most active and successful.

Council Goals and Effectiveness

The Scope of the Council's Substantive Interests

All official promulgations of the Council's purposes authorized the mechanism to explore the full range of relationships among the member agencies' programs.[12] Nevertheless, the Council usually concerned itself with a limited spectrum of the substantive relationships, as a brief review of several major questions concerning the distribution of responsibilities among these agencies reveals:

1. In New York as in many other states, mental health services and other areas of public health are separated departmentally, although the mentally ill usually have somatic needs and many persons receiving common medical services require psychiatric or related services. Nonetheless, the Council did relatively little to explore the broad relationships among the medical programs of the Departments of Mental Hygiene, Health, Social Welfare, and other departments. For example, it did little to evaluate and foster the integration of the services of these agencies so that clienteles might receive comprehensive and coordinated care.

2. The State Education Department provides vocational services and the Department of Labor employment services that are

11. To overcome the aforementioned obstacles would require a much more extensive research effort than is possible within the scope of this study. Furthermore, aside from the burden of assumptions that such an effort would have to bear, it is questionable that the research would yield knowledge commensurate with the effort involved.

12. See Notes 5, 6, and 7, above, for the references to the three official documents under which the Council operated.

needed by many persons with mental illness. Yet, the Council did not attempt to work out arrangements to ensure that persons discharged from the state's mental institutions receive, as needed, the vocational services offered by these agencies.

3. The Education Department has among its responsibilities the health education of school children. It therefore has an important effect on the understanding and attitudes of young people in matters of health. However, the Council was unable to act on this subject.

4. The Departments of Health and Social Welfare both have broad responsibilities for medical care and share overlapping clienteles. Nevertheless, there was no systematic examination in the Council of most of the points at which their programs met or converged.

5. The Council did not examine relationships between the environmental health functions of the Department of Health and the Department of Labor's responsibilities for the health of workers on and off the job.

The Council tended to focus its attention upon the problems of special population groups. As the names of its most active committees reveal, the Council dealt largely with the problems of serving the physically handicapped, chronic alcoholics, narcotics addicts, mentally retarded persons, especially children, emotionally disturbed children, and the aged. An analysis of the headings in the minutes of the Council during the IHRB and IHHC periods suggests that, except for procedural questions, matters involving these groups accounted for more than 65 percent of all of the subjects considered by the commissioners.[13]

The Types of Council Activity

The Council's purposes were characterized by such key concepts as: planning, cooperative study and action, program development, exchange of information, and interdepartmental consulta-

13. Such administrative and procedural matters as election of the chairman, review of minutes, reports by the agencies of their legislative plans, and discussion of plans for future meetings were excluded from the analysis.

tion, as the preceding quotations from the official documents partly illustrate.[14] Since these concepts imply that the Council was a decision-making structure (planning, program development, and cooperative study and action) and an instrument of interdepartmental communication (exchange of information, interdepartmental consultation, and cooperative study), it is appropriate to analyze the mechanism in terms of its performance of each of these basic objectives.

The Council as a decision-making structure. The Council was ineffective with respect to decision-making, for it was not basically a decision-making body. It did not systematically examine problems in their broad implications or decide on means and ends for dealing with them. Although the Council's committees conducted many useful studies, such efforts and any ensuing recommendations typically skirted sensitive and controversial issues. Moreover, for the Council the process of decision-making was ad hoc and exceedingly incremental. Most of the agenda items were questions that were brought up opportunistically by one or more members when they felt it advantageous to do so, and any action taken usually was slow in coming. For example, of the 64 rehabilitation issues brought before the Council after the formation of the Committee on Rehabilitation in 1953, including 12 that still were under consideration at the end of 1964, almost half were under consideration for more than two years, and more than one-fourth were still active issues after five years.[15]

Consequently, the Council did little to influence the basic goals and functions of its member agencies, even in the substantive areas in which it was most active, for the agencies regarded their constitutional and legislative underpinnings as sacrosanct. For example, the Council almost never recommended the transfer of functions from one agency to another. Of all rehabilitation issues to come before the mechanism, only 8 percent presented the pos-

14. See Notes 5, 6, and 7, above.

15. The procedures followed in classifying rehabilitation issues are described in the Appendix.

sibility of a transfer of functions (5 of 64), and the member agencies were unable to resolve any of these because they were highly controversial. Similarly, the member agencies usually avoided recommending legislation; benign support of each other's legislative aspirations, in instances of overall agreement, characterized the extent of their general involvement. For instance, although 30 percent of the rehabilitation issues presented the possibility of statutory change (19 of 64), the member agencies recommended action in only 3 percent of them (2 of 64).

The Council sometimes gave broad charges to its committees to review the relationships of agency programs, including the opportunity to make changes in the locus of responsibilities. For example, in 1954, the chairman of the Council requested the fledgling Committee on Rehabilitation

> to consider the constitutional responsibilities of the respective departments in . . . [the field of chronic disease] as well as departmental responsibilities in the administration of the pertinent federal programs and the allocation of federal funds under these programs . . . [to] facilitate the development of recommendations for a Statewide program, outlining the departmental functions and responsibilities and those functions which should be carried out on an interdepartmental basis.[16]

However, such charges were almost never fulfilled, owing to the agencies' need to protect their autonomy. As a result, the Council had little effect on the division of health responsibilities in the state, and it was not an important source of legislation.

Similarly, the Council was not a medium for systematically reviewing the agencies' needs for resources, establishing priorities, and recommending allocations. Consequently, it did not influence the basic allocation of resources among the state's health programs, that is, funds, manpower, and clients. Moreover, on the occasions that the Council attempted to advise with respect to such allocations, it was usually rebuffed. For example, when

16. Minutes of the IHC, March 23, 1954, p. 2.

the Council tried to persuade the Division of the Budget and the Civil Service Department to upgrade the salary scale for certain rehabilitation personnel that were in short supply, it apparently had no effect.[17] Yet, although the Council did not function as a resource-allocating mechanism, through its decisions it somewhat influenced the flow of resources among health programs. For example, the exchange of resources among the member agencies or between them and third parties, such as the Division of the Budget, was expected as a result of action taken in 75 percent of the rehabilitation issues on which some agreement was reached in the Council (27 of 37). Furthermore, some resources were in fact exchanged as a result of the Council's decisions, as will be shown.

The Council as an instrument of interdepartmental communication. In contrast to its ineffectiveness as a decision-making body, the Council was a rather effective instrument of interdepartmental communication. As has been amply demonstrated in the preceding chapters, most of its energies were devoted to exchanging information and points of view through discussion and study of questions of mutual interest. The informational activities of the Council were also of broader scope than its decision-making efforts, with member agencies exchanging information through the Council about such matters as impending state legislation, the actions of the governor and his aides, and significant developments on the national health scene. Consequently, the member agencies not only greatly increased their understanding of each other, but expanded their knowledge of the activities, points of view, and ambitions of the other organizations and groups. Furthermore, they learned much about the dimensions of health problems, such as the needs of particular groups, gaps in service, and the obstacles to providing effective services.

Yet, notwithstanding the fact that the Council ranged farther afield in communicating than in making decisions, it is important

17. See p. 63.

to recognize that these two activities usually went hand in hand and reinforced each other. Decision-making requires information, much of which is of value beyond the agreements for which it is requisite. Likewise, cooperative action usually leads to further exchange of information.

Finally, the Council's educational activities extended beyond its membership, such as to the governor, private health agencies, and professional associations, for the Council disseminated to others a considerable amount of information about health matters in the form of reports, articles, and letters, and verbally as well.

How Much Difference the Council Made

Another way of assessing the effect of the Council is to consider what actions have been taken as a result of its decisions—actions that otherwise would not likely have been taken (or would probably have been executed differently) if the Council had not made a decision. In other words, "decisive" as distinguished from "indecisive" efforts may well be identified. This is an exceedingly difficult, perhaps impossible, question to answer.[18] Nevertheless, there is enough evidence to make some reasonable estimates of the Council's impact.

The most striking aspect of the Council's impact is that there are relatively few programs or actions that would not have been accomplished, or would have been executed much differently, if the Council had not acted.[19] On most substantive matters the Council made it easier for the members to reach agreement and increased somewhat the likelihood that the objectives would be attained. Even in the area of rehabilitation, the program sector in which the instrumentality was most active and productive, the

18. This problem arises both because of the difficulty of determining what effects the Council had and what things would have been undertaken differently if it had not acted.

19. Excluded from consideration are the actions taken by the Council in conducting the research and demonstration projects for which it was responsible during the IHRB period.

Council's decisions seem to have been decisive in no more than one-fourth of the issues on which it took some action. Furthermore, wherever the Council had a decisive effect, its accomplishment was generally very modest. Insofar as the Council was a decision-making body, the member agencies used it mainly to work out minor revisions in their policies and procedures, and to help convince governors and other principals to make small changes in state policies, to expand existing programs, and support the development of new ones.

The limited effect of the instrumentality as a decisional structure can be demonstrated most convincingly through examples of Council decisions that have had the most decisive and broadest consequences. Again, the area of rehabilitation, in which the Council functioned at its best, provides the most applicable illustrations.

An excellent example of decisive action is the part played by the Council in the development of the Workshop Support Program administered by the Division of Vocational Rehabilitation of the State Education Department. This episode also illustrates the drawn-out character of the decision-making process. In 1957, the Council received from a group of influential executives of voluntary agencies several communications critical of the adequacy of the state's vocational rehabilitation services. These letters stimulated interest in the financial plight and special needs of sheltered workshops, which are facilities that employ and train physically handicapped persons. The result was that a subcommittee of the Committee on Rehabilitation was set up to study the needs of the shops. Subsequently, over a two-year period questionnaires were sent to workshops throughout the state. Members of the subcommittee visited a number of facilities, and the possibility of recommending that the state provide financial support to needy shops, most of which are voluntary nonprofit organizations, was carefully considered. However, it was decided that the time was not propitious for action, because the workshop field was in the throes of developing standards. The response of the workshops generally had been negative, and the data that had been collected did not present a case convincing enough to justify recommendations for a new program. There also were some underlying jealousies and tensions among the agencies about which department should have responsibility for a new program.

However, although the Council did not then act, its study of workshops generated further interest in the problem, both in and out of state government, which spread to the Governor's Council on Rehabilitation and to the governor's office. Eventually the climate became more favorable for action. In 1960, the Council reactivated its subcommittee on workshops and helped to formulate the Workshop Support Program, which Governor Rockefeller accepted in 1962. The program finally was implemented in 1964 after a number of legislative and appropriation hurdles were overcome. Subsequently, the Council, through the Committee on Rehabilitation, continued to provide counsel to the Education Department on the administration of the program.

Although the Council played a major part in the development of the new program, it is by no means certain that the program would not have come into being anyway. The Department of Education and the Governor's Council on Rehabilitation were pressing for action, and the earlier establishment of the Rehabilitation Center Program gave impetus to doing something for sheltered workshops.[20] Nevertheless, it seems that the Council

20. Some may feel that the Council's involvement in the Rehabilitation Center Program should have been presented as a decisive action. Although the existence of the Council and its interest in rehabilitation awakened the interest of the governor's staff in developing the program, this consequence was entirely fortuitous and not a direct result of Council action. The member of the governor's office who drafted the program got his inspiration while studying the Council in connection with the Rockefeller reorganization of the executive branch. The Rehabilitation Center Program also was prepared by the governor's aide in unilateral discussions with representatives of most of the agencies belonging to the Committee on Rehabilitation as well as with others, and not through the Council. The Council was brought into the matter only after the program had been formulated and the decision to go ahead had been made. Furthermore, as shown in the previous chapter, although the Council, particularly the Committee on Rehabilitation,

had some influence on the outcome, for it not only helped to generate and shape much of the interest in developing the Workshop Program, but it mustered valuable technical assistance as well. Certainly, such a program as might have been developed without the Council would have taken longer to activate and probably would have been different. An official of the Education Department who was intimately acquainted with the development of the program said, "If there had not been a Council it would have been harder to get it across. It was the general interest, support, and availability of the Council that gave strength to the proposal and got it adopted."

In another instance of decisive action, the Council was responsible for a change in state policy that might not otherwise have been made; however, the action was very modest. In the early 1960's, the member agencies began a series of deliberations that eventually led to gubernatorial action to make public buildings accessible to severely handicapped persons. This series of events began when a member of Governor Rockefeller's staff received a letter from the wife of a prominent university dean who was a victim of polio, pointing out how disabled persons could maintain their independence through various adaptations made in public buildings. The aide forwarded the letter to the Council, suggesting that it be distributed to the departments that might be interested. The request fell upon receptive ears, for the Council decided to study the matter itself through its Committee on Rehabilitation, and about a year later recommended that the Governor take appropriate action to require that all public buildings have doors sufficiently wide to accommodate wheel chairs, grade-level entrances or ramps, appropriate toilet facilities, and other features to alleviate the problem. As a result, in July, 1961, Governor Rockefeller issued a directive making it a state policy that all new state buildings meet appropriate standards. This set

helped in the implementation of the program, it did not play a decisive role. The decisions that it helped to make would have been made by the Department of Health anyway and they probably would not have been made much differently.

in motion a series of subsequent efforts at the gubernatorial level and within the state departments to implement the new policy. The Council also continued to exhibit considerable interest in the matter and to exert its influence in various ways. For example, it kept an eye on the pace of implementation, prodded for more effective action, and recommended legislation to expand the policy to municipalities. Yet, even though the Council played a major role in the development of what is considered a most enlightened state policy toward the handicapped, and probably a decisive one, it is by no means certain that the groups that were pushing for state action would not have eventually succeeded, for the climate of opinion generally was favorable. A key participant in the issue commented, "It would have happened anyway, but the fact of the matter is it happened there [in the Council]. The Council facilitated and probably speeded up the process . . . it acted as a catalyst."

The Council also seems to have had a fairly decisive role in changes made by the Education Department in its policies for licensing physical therapists. This activity, however, also illustrated the incremental character and slow pace of Council decision-making. The issue, which was on and off the agenda for over a decade, concerned the adverse effect of state licensing policies upon the supply of physical therapists in New York. Many charged that these policies, which were the most rigid in the nation, made it extremely difficult to recruit therapists. Consequently, during the life of the issue, most of the member agencies of the Council were under growing pressure from various medical and other groups, including the therapists themselves, to correct rigidities in the state's licensing program. Moreover, several of the Council agencies, such as the Department of Mental Hygiene, also were hard hit by the shortage of physical therapists, and thus were interested in change.

When the matter was first raised in the Council in 1953, following complaints from a prominent physician who directed a rehabilitation facility, a physical therapist, to obtain a license, had to be a graduate of a school whose program was approved by the

State Education Department. If not, he was required to pass a special examination that was open only to those with equivalent education. For various reasons many could not qualify. Most of the nation's schools were not approved, including many certified by the American Medical Association's Committee on Medical Education. The schools also were expected to apply for approval, which some refused to do. Moreover, the requirements for admission to the special examination were vague, and the applicants who were rejected usually were not told why they had been turned down. Furthermore, a therapist qualified in another jurisdiction could not work in New York while waiting to be licensed.

The Council, however, approached the problem cautiously, for the unit of the State Education Department that licensed professional personnel was extremely reluctant to alter its policies and procedures. On several occasions the Education Department was asked to present its views—for example, when criticisms of state policy were made by influential citizens. Several studies of the problem were undertaken, which revealed, among other deficiencies, the seriousness of the shortage of therapists, and which pointed up the differences between the educational requirements in New York and elsewhere. In 1955, when the issue was especially intense, the Council formally recommended specific changes in Education Department policies, with the concurrence of the Commissioner of Education, who generally was more responsive to the outside pressures than the unit in his department responsible for professional licensing. Finally, under sustained pressure, both inside and outside of the Council, the Department gradually changed its policies and procedures. Thus by 1964, when the last obstacle to reshaping these policies was removed by legislative action, the critics generally were satisfied that a flexible and enlightened policy had been achieved.

Today the Education Department actively seeks to approve all schools of physical therapy that can qualify, and in certifying them, relies heavily on American Medical Association standards. Moreover, any graduate of a school certified by the Association who must take the special examination may practice in New York for a reasonable time while awaiting licensing. Even those persons lacking certain required courses are permitted to practice temporarily until they are able to make up their deficiencies, a policy which has helped to attract foreign as well as American therapists to New York.

The difficult question to answer is how much of a difference the Council made in these changes. Certainly the Council could not have acted in the absence of the outside pressures to which the member agencies, in particular the Education Department, were subjected. The Council's principal contribution seems to have come from focusing pressures on the State Education Department and giving the Commissioner of Education some needed support in moving the unit of his Department that was responsible for the licensing of professionals. This is the view of many knowledgeable state officials and private citizens, including representatives of the Education Department.

The occasion, cited earlier, in which the Council called for the development within the Department of Mental Hygiene of special services for emotionally disturbed blind children is a more clear-cut instance of decisive action taken under pressure. In mitigating the pressures generated by a private study that was severely critical of the adequacy of state services for these unfortunate children, the member agencies recommended that two new facilities be created, a program which reached fruition when Governor Rockefeller acted favorably upon the Council's proposal. Although the pressures in the situation probably would have resulted in some kind of state response if the Council had not acted, by focusing the pressures on the Department of Mental Hygiene, the Council made it more likely that the recommendations to which the Department very reluctantly agreed would be made and acted upon. According to a top official of the Department of Mental Hygiene who represented the Department at the time, the Council "provided a vehicle by which other agencies were able to exert pressure on the Department and get through to the governor's office." In his view the outcome would have been different if the issue had not been handled by the Council.

Two additional examples of decisive action further demonstrate the limited impact of the Council's decisions. In the first, the Council was instrumental in the establishment in the Department of Correction of a pilot center to serve epileptic prisoners. The issue first came before the Council in 1956, when the Correction Department invited the Committee on Rehabilitation to look into the needs for rehabilitation of physically handicapped prisoners. Following this request the Committee undertook a study in which the personnel of several departments participated. About two years later the Council approved recommendations aimed at strengthening the medical and rehabilitation services of the Department, one of which called for a pilot program to help epileptics. In the two years that followed, after a change in administration, and after the Governor's Council on Rehabilitation gave strong support to the recommendations, the governor's office decided to fund the proposal for the project for epileptics. In this instance the Council clearly formulated and gave essential support to a project that probably would not otherwise have come into being, as there was little impetus for any kind of action, even within the Department of Correction, until after the Council had issued its recommendations. In fact, as already indicated,[21] the Department considered the recommendations to be low in priority and thus did not welcome the growing support which sprang from various quarters.

In another instance, the Council helped to clear up conflicting policies regarding the provision of physical therapy services by proprietary nursing homes. The Departments of Health and Social Welfare advocated that such services be made available in nursing homes in pursuance of their philosophy of rehabilitation. However, a controversy arose when the Education Department interpreted state law to mean that proprietary, in contrast to nonprofit, homes were prohibited from employing physical therapists and advertising the availability of their services. After a representative of the Department of Health brought up the

21. See pp. 71–72.

matter, a subcommittee of the Committee on Rehabilitation was formed to investigate. This committee, with cooperation from the legal counsel of the Education Department, worked out a satisfactory interpretation, which permitted proprietary nursing homes to make physical therapy services available on their premises and to advertise them, provided they were paid for directly by the patient and prescribed by the patient's physician. The issue was resolved about eight months from the date it was born, when the Council accepted the Committee's report and authorized the Departments of Health and Social Welfare to distribute it as they saw fit. Clearly the Council moved with reasonable dispatch in this matter and the combined efforts of the member agencies probably helped to convince the Education Department that it should revise its interpretation of state law. Yet how much of a difference the Council made in the outcome is hard to say.

There are other Council decisions concerning rehabilitation services that are noteworthy, including several as influential as those already described, and some that may have had greater impact. However, most of the instances of Council decision not described here tend to have been indecisive and narrow in impact. It is largely a matter of degree and interpretation.

Moreover, there should be no inference that because the Council accomplished so little as a decision-making body that its decisions were not beneficial. Although the benefits were limited, considering the Council's two-decade history, they were nonetheless real and are recognized and acknowledged by many of the persons who have participated in Council activities.

Why the Council Was Not More Effective

The Council was not more effective, particularly as a decision-making body, because its member agencies were so readily threatened by any examination of the major relationships among their health responsibilities. They dared not risk going to the heart of most of the questions that were presented for Council deliberation. To face issues more squarely would either place the members in open competition for functions, resources, and prestige, or create the risk that conflict might break out among them. Even though the member agencies felt much freer to exchange information and views than to agree on joint action, because it is less threatening to do so, there were limits to this activity as well. Moreover, even if the Council were to have come to grips with controversial issues it could not have counted on the outside support needed to implement its decisions. Thus, given the inherent operating characteristics of the instrumentality and the inclination of New York governors to leave it alone, the Council could not have been more effective than it was. The Department of Health's lack of success in its vigorous efforts to bring forth crucial issues dividing the members is ample evidence that this is true. Consequently, the Council played little part in shaping major changes in the state's health programs during the two decades it existed.

But why did the Council focus its attention upon the problems of serving such special population groups as emotionally disturbed children, alcoholics, and the physically handicapped? Although several factors are relevant, in the main these program sectors represented fewer risks to the member agencies as cooperative endeavors; also they are areas in which pressures for coordination were greater. The risks of cooperating were lower, better known, and apparently easier to calculate, principally because limited segments of the agencies' total health responsibilities were involved. In addition, although the individual agencies regarded these areas as having varying importance to their programs, the special population groups generally represented peripheral activities for Council members. For example, the issues arising out of the relationships between the responsibilities of the Department of Mental Hygiene for the mentally ill and those of the Department of Social Welfare for the medically indigent were at the very heart of these agencies' functions; in contrast, the relationships between them in dealing with alcoholics and the physically handicapped were much less vital.

The Council members were also under greater outside pressure, largely indirect, to cooperate in meeting the problems of the special population groups than in fulfilling their broader responsibilities. This largely reflects the way in which interest groups in the health field are arrayed and make themselves felt and also the way in which governors influenced the Council. With the exception of professional organizations and a few powerful associations representing facilities, such as the American Hospital Association, private interest groups in the health field tend to be organized around the needs of special categories of patients or clients, such as crippled children, persons with heart disease, the mentally retarded, and the aged. Even the federal health programs tend to reflect what is known in the field as "categorical interests." Moreover, inasmuch as the private interest groups and the federal agencies concerned with special populations have been especially active since World War II, Council agencies have been under considerable pressure to expand and improve their programs for special clienteles. New York governors also have been responsive to these trends, and thus, when they turned to the Council, they influenced it accordingly.

The impact of outside influences has been particularly marked in the area of rehabilitation, which helps to explain why the Council was more active and productive in this program sector than in any others. During much of the life of the Council, private interest groups were especially active in rehabilitation and the growth of federal programs having an impact upon the state was far-reaching. Moreover, the Rockefeller administration referred more rehabilitation questions to the Council than did its predecessors, for the Governor had a strong personal interest in this area. And, as has been mentioned, the Governor's Council on Rehabilitation, set up in 1959 in response to influential private interests, became a source of gentle and friendly pressure upon the Council and the administration.

The Council agencies also needed each other's assistance most in serving special populations because they are among the most difficult groups to help. Usually they require special services and in many instances programs are minimal, as in the case of alcoholics and narcotics addicts, because knowledge is undeveloped. Furthermore, during much of the life of the Council, the agencies' responsibilities for these groups tended to be less clear and their programs less well developed than in other areas of concern.

CHAPTER 9

Alternatives and Conclusions

CONSIDERING the Council's difficulty in coordinating its members, one may wonder whether the agencies can be coordinated beyond what has been achieved by instrumentalities in the past—the governor, the Division of the Budget, the Council, etc.—and which, if any, of the alternatives to the council mechanism is preferable. To answer the questions posed, it seems desirable (1) to suggest criteria for selecting alternatives to the council mechanism; (2) to consider, as an alternative to the council mechanism, coordination of its members by hierarchy; and (3) to consider two specific alternatives to the council mechanism, including how its ability to coordinate might have been increased by changes in its structural constraints.

Evaluating the Alternatives to the Council Mechanism

It is impossible to specify the most suitable alternative to the council mechanism, whether it be a reorganized Council or another form of organization, without first deciding the extent to which the health programs of the state need to be coordinated. Although assessment of the coordinating capabilities of alternative structures is an essential step, the central question is one of deciding what is to be achieved and then determining how the programs of each agency need to be concerted to attain the desired objectives. Ideally, what type, or types, of coordination would be the most appropriate cannot be ascertained without an extensive evaluation of the state's health programs. Such an effort is necessary to decide both what kind of state program is needed as well as how it may best be realized. To do anything less would be to prescribe a remedy without the benefit of a diagnosis, a not infrequent course in organizational affairs. But if results under such circumstances are good, the outcome usually is a happy accident.

Obviously then, it is not possible in this study to make a final determination of what type of coordination is needed in New York. Because of the magnitude of the task it is not even possible to describe the health system of the state, or any major portion of it, let alone to evaluate the system or suggest a better one. To analyze what is a $650 million operation would require a team of specialists.[1]

What then can be said here? First, it is possible to consider briefly what kind of (ideal) study would be required to identify optimum coordination, including the limits of such a venture. Second, although it is not possible here to establish the empirical consequences of the alternatives to the council mechanism, it is important to explore their logical differences. This too should be useful to officials who, once having defined the need for coordination in a particular situation, must choose among several alternative structures. It also should be of interest to students of organization who are concerned with the theoretical issues.

A Systems Analysis of Health Activities in New York

Since the reason for coordinating the state's health activities is to increase through joint decision-making the extent to which, and the efficiency with which, certain objectives are achieved, the most promising way of determining how much and what kind of coordination is essential is to analyze the health programs of the

1. See pp. 36–37.

state as a system of related parts. This approach has the advantage of focusing attention upon both the connections among the programs and their place in the overall health effort of the state. Such a study should include the following basic steps: (1) specification of the system and program objectives to be achieved; (2) assessment of how well these goals are being attained presently; (3) consideration of alternative ways of accomplishing the objectives, including the benefits and costs of each alternative; and (4) identification of the kind of organizational arrangements that seem most appropriate to each alternative, and hence the type of coordination that seems most suitable.

Scope of the study. Depending upon the magnitude and importance of the questions to be examined, the study might encompass all or part of the health responsibilities of the executive branch. Since these dimensions may not be known in advance, one approach is to begin with the most significant health functions—for example, with the programs of the core agencies—and to enlarge the study if the results suggest that expansion is desirable. Thus, for instance, if it is found that the programs of the core departments and some of the other agencies are closely linked, the scope of the study might be expanded. Another approach is to begin with problem areas, such as with state responsibilities for dealing with chronic alcoholism and narcotics addiction.

Definition of program goals. Since the type of coordination that may be required is a function of what is to be achieved, a primary step is to define the objectives of the system or subsystem being analyzed and each of its component programs. Program objectives are, however, typically stated in general terms and usually are difficult if not impossible to formulate precisely. Also it is common that programs have multiple goals. Consequently, defining goals usually means deciding on what they shall be. Clearly this requires the participation of policy-making officials; a system's analysis is not a neutral endeavor. Since the major purpose of mapping the system and its component programs is to provide a basis for making choices, it is important that programs and their objectives be defined in a manner that will facilitate comparison of alternatives. It is desirable, for example, to know whether any programs may be viewed as substitutes for others.

Achievement of program goals. One cannot choose among alternative means of pursuing desired objectives without having a reasonably good idea of how well existing programs meet these objectives. But, as already discussed, organizational effectiveness is exceedingly difficult to measure, for both methodological and technical reasons.[2] At best the analysis will have to rely largely upon indices from which the programs' effectiveness can be inferred, and hence upon such measures as the number and kind of persons served and the number of units of service provided. Policy officials, therefore, should participate in the formulation and interpretation of such measures. It is particularly important to try to develop criteria that facilitate comparison of the outputs of existing and substitute programs, such as financial data and quantitative measures of output.

Evaluation of alternatives. Given agreement on the objectives to be achieved and a reasonable estimation of the effectiveness of existing programs, it is necessary that the benefits and costs of alternative ways of achieving these goals be considered. There is, of course, almost no limit in principle to the number of alternatives that could be considered. The practical limit will depend upon the characteristics of the program sector being scrutinized and the scope and depth of the analysis. In general, however, only those alternatives that appear to promise meaningful benefits should be examined. For example, the goals of mental health may better be served through the use of varied technologies and professional skills, or by different organizational arrangements of existing technologies and skills. Would group work supervised by clinical psychologists in contrast to individual therapy provided by psychiatrists, or a new combination of these approaches, be the most practical and effective way of rehabilitating the mentally ill? Similarly, would the health needs of school children be better

2. See pp. 183–87.

and/or less expensively served by assigning the responsibility to public health officials instead of to educational authorities? Would services to crippled children be carried out better by state-operated services or by grants-in-aid to local government agencies or to private groups? Would a policy of requiring the relatives of some clients, if they are able, to pay part of the costs of the medical services furnished contribute to or distract from state goals?

In evaluating existing as well as alternative programs, it is essential to consider how the programs impinge upon each other, both to ascertain the advantages and disadvantages of different program arrangements and determine what organizational relationships would seem most appropriate for them. Consequently, it is important to raise such questions as these: To what extent is the output of one program an input of another? For example, the patients discharged by the Department of Mental Hygiene may be inputs of the Division of Vocational Rehabilitation of the State Education Department and the Employment Service of the Department of Labor. The nature of these relationships may suggest the need for closer relationships among the programs of these agencies. Do any of the programs overlap, and, if so, do they complement or duplicate each other? For instance, the Division of Vocational Rehabilitation and the Employment Service both help handicapped workers find employment. Whether these programs complement each other, as they seem to do, or wastefully duplicate each other may indicate whether or not they should be merged. To what extent are any of the programs alternatives to each other, so that if one is expanded the need for another would be reduced? To illustrate, some of the environmental health and research programs of the Department of Health may diminish the need for certain medical care programs of the Department of Social Welfare, as for example the services it provides to persons having communicable diseases. Similarly, expansion of the enrollment in the professional schools of the State University may reduce the need for the professional manpower recruitment programs of the other agencies. And finally, in instances in which changes in one program affect another, how long does it take for the impact to be felt? Thus, whether a research program may be expected to have immediate or long-range effects may be a factor in deciding how to plan for changes in related programs.

Identification of appropriate organizational arrangements. The last step of the study is to decide which mix of programs will achieve the desired goals at least cost or maximize goal attainment for a given cost. The study should provide a good idea of how much and in what ways the programs selected need to be coordinated, if at all. Depending upon the requirements of the system and its component parts, various kinds of coordination may be called for. Thus, for example, in some areas programs might need to be merged or reassigned among the agencies, or a wholly new department may be required. In other sectors, it may be desirable to create a "czar" in the governor's office to concert the programs. And in still others, little or no coordination may be required. Furthermore, where coordination may be necessary, the type needed may vary. In some areas it may be sufficient to coordinate program-planning activities. In others it may be enough to coordinate the implementation of programs, such as the referral of patients from one agency to another. Then again some situations may require both kinds. Moreover, the type of coordination that is most appropriate in a particular situation may change as circumstances change. Consequently, it may be desirable to reexamine and define the need for coordination periodically.

This ideal study would be a very difficult undertaking. The problem in defining program goals and measuring the output of organizations already has been mentioned.[3] There also are serious technical problems in acquiring the information needed to conduct a systems analysis. But much more fundamental, the extent to which program objectives can be specified and effective ways of realizing them identified in any policy sector depends upon how well defined are the problems involved and whether there

3. See pp. 183–87.

are clear solutions to them. If there is not a sufficient body of reliable knowledge on the nature of these problems and how they can be attacked, there will be inadequate criteria for making decisions on any basis other than individual judgment. Consequently, the degree to which there is uncertainty and disagreement among specialists on how to deal with health problems will limit how far it is possible to define objectively the organizational, and thus the coordinative needs, of the system. Moreover, the maintenance and enhancement needs of the agencies and others must be taken into account in choosing the program objectives and in selecting the ways to pursue them, for these needs cannot be suspended while the need for coordination is being diagnosed.[4] Nevertheless, notwithstanding its limitations, such a systematic and self-conscious effort is essential if the need for coordination among health programs in New York is to be determined objectively. If to coordinate these programs means to increase the rationality by which they are directed, one must confront the questions that have been posed. That the questions rarely are confronted is the reason why most discussions of coordination are so empty—lip service is paid to a vague, and largely meaningless, desideratum.

Although this is the ideal, scientific, and logical way of determining how much coordination is needed among particular programs, obviously it is not a practical approach, and one that is unlikely to be tried. The time and effort required to implement such determination would be considerable, to say nothing of the difficulties of mastering the intellectual problems that are involved. Recognizing this, and bearing in mind that such an

4. For a discussion of the applicability to nonmilitary sectors of the federal government, including health, of program budgeting and systems analysis techniques developed in the Department of Defense, see David Novick, ed., *Program Budgeting* (Cambridge, Mass., 1965), esp. pp. 3–60 and 208–47. Two other good discussions of the application of such techniques in government are found in Roland N. McKean, *Efficiency in Government through Systems Analysis* (New York, 1958), and Charles J. Hitch and Roland N. McKean, *The Economics of Defense in the Nuclear Age* (New York, 1965; originally published Cambridge, Mass. 1960).

approach nevertheless offers the only scientific basis for diagnosing the need for coordination, the next step is to consider alternative coordinating mechanisms. Accordingly, the alternatives are examined with a view to their potential effect upon relations among the agencies, rather than their effect in increasing coordination of programs or areas of health responsibility.

Coordination by Hierarchy

Of the two principal types of coordination—coordination by council and by hierarchy—this study presents strong evidence that the former is ineffective when the reconciliation of agency differences is an important consideration. Generally a council is able to concert the activities of its members only to the extent that they can cooperate voluntarily, or in effect, when it is in the interest of the agencies to coordinate themselves. A council is powerless to do otherwise, and the governor and others have not expected it to be more effective. Any attempt, therefore, substantially to increase coordination of the agencies would have to make use of hierarchical elements.[5] This makes it important, before considering the specific alternatives to the council mechanism, to examine the logic of greater hierarchical coordination.

One way of exploring the hierarchical alternative to the council mechanism is to consider how a powerful "czar" set up in its place would change the situation. Presenting a polar case has the advantage of setting in relief the principal characteristics of the alternative. Since the czar is merely a device for exploring the coordinating power of the alternatives to the council mechanism, no effort is made here to consider how he would affect the main institutions of the state government, such as the governor and the legislature; however, it seems best to imagine the czar as being the governor, or someone responsible to him.

5. This study has been concerned with "managed" as distinguished from "unmanaged" coordination. See pp. 9–10.

The Conditions Necessary for Coordination

To coordinate the agencies perfectly would require drastic centralization of the authority that they now possess, as it is the extensive division of labor among them and their units and the considerable discretion that the agencies enjoy that gives rise both to the ostensible need for coordination and the obstacles to achieving it. As with many large bureaucratic organizations, the departments are characterized by extensive specialization of work and decentralization of decision-making. Witness the great variety and number of highly trained professionals—physicians, educators, nurses, therapists, social workers, engineers, etc.—and semi-professionals upon which the agencies depend to meet their responsibilities. Extensive specialization and delegation of authority, however, increases the interdependence of the units within each agency and of the agencies themselves, and thereby increases the demand for intradepartmental and interdepartmental coordination. Similarly, by increasing the number of interdependent agencies and departmental subgroups, specialization and delegation also add to the difficulties of achieving both types of coordination, for each of the agencies and their subgroups develop maintenance and enhancement needs based upon their special views and their desire to remain autonomous.[6] This leads to competition among the agencies and their units for scarce resources—such as funds, manpower, clients, and status—and consequently a resistance to coordination.[7]

The Benefits and Costs of Coordination

A czar presumably could solve the problems of coordination, for through his authority and power he could control the divisive

6. Philip Selznick has shown how the delegation of authority leads to division of interests and conflict among the subunits of an organization that is dysfunctional for achievement of the organization's goals. See *TVA and The Grass Roots* (Berkeley, 1953).

7. The specific need for coordination and the specific obstacles to it of course change with changes in such areas as medical technology, concepts of health service, public pressures for services, and internal and external shifts in agency responsibilities. New issues therefore are always being generated and old ones change.

forces among the agencies. By making the costs of resisting coordination significantly high he could compel the agencies and their units to face up to differences and make the necessary changes in policies and procedures to coordinate their programs. Moreover, a czar would be immune to the play of political forces upon and through the agencies. To the extent of his power he would contain and overshadow these forces.

The centralization of authority required to coordinate the agencies perfectly, however, would be costly. First, it would cause a decline in the professional esprit of agency personnel, although this would be counterbalanced somewhat by the ability of the czar in commanding the agencies to adopt and implement new ideas. Greater centralization also would increase organizational rigidities, and thus its accompanying dysfunctions. In addition, it would make it much more difficult to get public support for state health programs. Finally, it is doubtful that a czar could make decisions of greater benefit to the people of New York than are now possible through the governor and other existing instrumentalities.

Perhaps the greatest loss would be a decline in the competence of the agencies' professional members, which would have adverse implications for their performance and thus for accomplishment of the agencies' responsibilities. Tight reining of the agencies and their subgroups would impoverish the incentives by which they are able to induce persons to become organization members, and, once a part of the organization, to contribute their time and skills to the tasks at hand. Mainly, it would deprive the agencies of the ability to offer their members, particularly professional workers, considerable independence in their work. But it would be an extremely harmful deprivation, for the freedom that professional workers customarily enjoy in applying the canons of their profession to their work and the status that this brings them as members of their organization and profession are among their most important gratifications.[8] Any diminution in the availability

8. Peter M. Blau and W. Richard Scott note that "one of the central issues in contemporary professional organizations . . . is the conflict between

of these incentives therefore would make it more difficult for the departments to recruit essential staff and encourage outstanding work from their members. This consequence would be further reinforced because the agencies would tend to attract and retain persons with a high tolerance for authority and a low identification with their profession.[9] Such persons therefore would be among the less competent members of their profession.

The centralization of authority and resources among the agencies also would have the paradoxical effect of decreasing the creativity of their personnel while at the same time increasing the agencies' abilities as organizations to implement new ideas acceptable to the czar.[10] As to the first, the agencies' personnel, because of the cutback in freedom to exercise one's judgment, would lose incentives to conceive and propose new ideas. Furthermore, by specifying work tasks more precisely, a central authority would further dry up the wellsprings of innovation, for organization members would have fewer opportunities to be creative. On the other hand, the chances that the agencies could adopt innovative proposals acceptable to the czar would be increased because the centralization of authority would make it much easier to overcome internal resistance to change.

disciplined compliance with administrative procedures and adherence to professional standards in the performance of duties." See *Formal Organizations* (San Francisco, 1962), p. 36.

9. To use Alvin W. Gouldner's distinction, the proportion of "locals" to "cosmopolitans" would increase, or "those high on loyalty to the employing organization, low on commitment to specialized role skills, and likely to use an inner reference group orientation," compared with "those low on loyalty to the employing organization, high on commitment to specialized role skills, and likely to use outer reference group orientation." See "Toward an Analysis of Latent Social Roles, I and II," *Administrative Science Qtly.*, II (Dec. 1957 and March 1959), pp. 281–306 and 444–80.

10. The argument here rests heavily upon views expressed by James Q. Wilson, who has hypothesized that "the greater the diversity of the organization (in either its incentive system or its task structure or both), the *greater* the likelihood that some members will *conceive* major innovations, the *greater* the likelihood some members will *propose* innovations, and the *less* likelihood that the organization will *adopt* the innovations." See "Innovation in Organization: Notes Toward a Theory," in *Approaches to Organizational Design*, ed. James D. Thompson (Pittsburgh, 1966), pp. 195–218.

Curbing the agencies and their units would also require greater reliance upon such central devices as rules and close supervision, in contrast to delegation of authority. To insure that coordinated efforts would be carried out would demand much greater use of rules, or standard operating procedures. But, as Robert Merton has shown, when rules are relied upon heavily, they tend to become accepted by organization members as ends in themselves, which interferes with accomplishment of the purposes that the rules were designed to serve.[11] The rigidities and impersonalism that rules produce can only increase the difficulty that an organization has in satisfying its clients, an especially serious consequence for agencies providing health services. In addition, close supervision not only tends to increase tension in work groups, but when applied to professional personnel, who have high status and ego needs, and who are usually accorded a degree of autonomy, it also is particularly likely to evoke behavior that is undesirable from the point of view of the organization—for example, an unwillingness to work at a high level of productivity.[12]

By reducing the opportunities of private interest groups to influence state policy, centralizing authority in the hands of a czar also would make it harder to gain public support for the agencies' health programs. Private interest groups in the health field (such as client groups, professional associations, and voluntary health agencies) play a vital part in generating public support for their programs. In return, they expect to help shape state policies by exerting influence upon the organs of the state, including the legislature, the governor, and the agencies. However, since these groups characteristically represent special and parochial interests, such as the physically handicapped, hospitals, and pro-

11. Robert K. Merton, *Social Theory and Social Structure* (rev. ed.; New York, 1957), pp. 195–206.

12. In discussing individual's motivation to produce, James D. March and Herbert A. Simon argue: "If the maintenance of ego and status position is important to individuals, the more detailed the supervision the greater will be the number of alternatives evoked of a nonorganizational character [on the part of the employee]." See *Organizations* (New York, 1959), p. 55.

fessional associations, they constitute an impediment to interdepartmental coordination. In fact, to a significant extent the organization of the state's health functions reflects the organization and power of the interest groups active in the field. Consequently, in order to coordinate the agencies, a czar would have to limit sharply the opportunities of these groups to exert influence, thereby decreasing their activity and the likelihood of their being organized.

Moreover, if the agencies were perfectly coordinated, less attention probably would be given to special population groups, which would further reduce the level of public support. It is much harder to mobilize public interest and resources for broad health purposes, such as for improved medical care generally, than to meet the needs of particular groups, such as the handicapped, the medically indigent, and old people. The chance that private interest groups have to wield influence on behalf of their constituents is the price that is paid for the support such groups bring to health programs generally as well as particularly.

Finally, in addition to the stultifying effect that a czar would have upon the agencies, there also is serious doubt that he could make decisions more sound than those now being made in meeting the health needs of the people of New York, for his responsibility for making decisions probably would outrun his competence. Because of the magnitude and complexity of the problems with which he would have to deal, a czar would have enormous difficulty in deciding what to do. It also would be impossible for him to possess all of the technical expertise required to exercise sound judgment. He could, of course, overcome this difficulty somewhat by delegating much of his responsibility to subordinates, but this would produce among his subunits the kind of division of interests that gives rise to the demand for coordination. Furthermore, it is questionable that a real czar would try to live up to his position by making sweeping decisions regulating the relationships among the agencies to be coordinated. Because of the risks of making mistakes—the more comprehensive his decisions the greater the potential error—a real czar probably would be circumspect and cautious. But this would tend to vitiate the justification for his existence.

The reason for exploring the logic of a czar is not that it is a practical approach. There would be little if any support for it, and enormous opposition. The reason for considering a czar is to show that there is no way of achieving greater coordination without paying a price. The problem is one of optimizing competing values, mainly the benefits of concerting the agencies' health activities and the advantages of delegating authority to specialists.[13] Bearing this in mind, it is appropriate to turn to more modest ways of increasing coordination.

Two Alternatives to the Council Mechanism

Although the fact is usually not recognized in the literature of public administration, much of the competition and conflict among the agencies may be fairly well coordinated in an unmanaged fashion through the various ways by which the agencies adjust and adapt to each other's policies—by processes that Charles Lindblom calls "mutual adjustment."[14] As Lindblom observes:

> Paradoxically, preoccupation with central coordination may encourage one to underestimate the magnitude of the task of coordination, even to form a misconception of the nature of the process. The task of coordination is often identified with that part of it which is in

13. As Blau and Scott observe, "An implicit assumption of bureaucratic theory . . . is that hierarchical authority and discipline are compatible with decisions based on expert judgments made in accordance with professional standards. It seems, on the contrary, that there is conflict between these two conditions. Rigid discipline stifles professional judgments. Conversely, hierarchical authority is weakened by increasing technological complexity in an organization with its resulting emphasis on technical expertness for all personnel, including those on the lowest levels." See Blau and Scott, p. 185.

14. The subsequent discussion rests heavily on views recently enunciated by Charles E. Lindblom in *The Intelligence of Democracy* (New York, 1965). The processes that Lindblom calls "mutual adjustment" are those that occur among partisans (decision-makers who make decisions calculated to serve their own goals, not goals presumably shared by other decision-makers with whom they are interdependent, except as they are controlled by other partisans or by central supervision), as distinguished from

fact attacked through central coordination; what [be]comes clear on second thought is forgotten—that an enormous amount of coordination is inevitably achieved through various mutual adjustments. But the most visible part of the coordination iceberg, explicit central coordination, may be only a small part of all those processes through which coordination to a degree is achieved.[15]

Lindblom recently has shown that these processes, which include such responses as one agency deferring to another, negotiating, bargaining, and partisan discussion, perform a valuable function in coordinating differences among organizations that is not necessarily inferior to coordination by a central decision-maker.[16] Far from necessarily sacrificing the interests of the people of New York to individual departmental points of view, the mutual adjustments that the agencies make may result in even sounder decisions, especially when there is not a clear standard by which to judge the public interest. For instance, these mutual adjustments not only are likely to insure that most if not all relevant points of view are reflected in state policy, but common values are more likely to emerge from the accompanying clash of ideas than from central decision-making.[17] Lindblom also argues that the decisions resulting from mutual adjustments are less likely to be in error. Moreover, when they are undesirable, they usually are more easily corrected, for in being adaptive, such decision-making is incremental.

cooperative decision-making among decision-makers acting in a nonpartisan way. "Mutual adjustment is defined as partisan not to contrast it with the ordinary case of central coordination of subordinate decision makers by a coordinating and separate decision maker . . . but specifically to contrast it with the case of decision makers who cooperatively (in a non-partisan way) constitute themselves collectively a coordinating decision maker" (pp. 21–34).

15. *Ibid.*, p. 170.

16. In Lindblom's definition, "a set of decisions is coordinated if adjustments have been made in it such that the adverse consequences of any one decision for other decisions in the set are to a degree and in some frequency avoided, reduced, counterbalanced, or outweighed" (*ibid.*, p. 154).

17. As Lindblom says, "the special interests can utilize, discipline, and curb each other to achieve, among other things, a more general interest" (*ibid.*, p. 302).

Processes of mutual adjustment also play an indispensable part in making a system of managed coordination work. To illustrate: the governor does not attempt to settle through decision each of the policy disagreements among his departments. For one thing, there frequently are no clear criteria available by which to judge the merits of these issues, and thus the public interest in the matter. For another, the governor lacks the technical expertise and often the information to evaluate competing claims. And, of course, he may lack the power to act without having to pay too high a price. The configuration of his authority and power, however, constitute a framework within which the processes of mutual adjustment among the contending agencies operate, a framework that gives weight to some values and not to others. It is also a framework that in varying degrees the governor is able to shape, and thereby he can influence the outcome of issues. But the governor rarely decides the issues in question, except when a resolution has sufficiently matured that he can strategically and advantageously exercise the authority of his office. Instead the governor usually is the key actor in and manipulator of the process of bureaucratic politics. A former member of Governor Rockefeller's staff seemed to acknowledge this when he reported, "The governor has no trouble supervising 200 agencies. . . . Every agency has a group of pressure groups in it; if they are in fairly close balance the governor feels things are fairly well coordinated."

The problem of how much the agencies need to be coordinated, therefore, probably can best be approached by asking the question: What things need to be coordinated centrally, and what things may be left to processes of mutual adjustment, or if you will, to politics? Although this question certainly cannot be answered here (the kind of study that has been already suggested is necessary), it seems that to increase coordination modest changes are probably needed in existing hierarchical arrangements, or the use of managerial strategies that will channel the political process in ways that will capitalize on its assets. There are a range of such alternatives to the council mechanism, which vary in their advantages and disadvantages; no way exists, however, of determining with reasonable certainty what arrangements will optimize the desired values. The state of organizational knowledge is too crude for that.

Two alternatives are briefly explored in the remainder of this chapter—a managerial strategy, and a reformed council.[18] The argument rests heavily upon the findings presented in the previous chapters and logical exploration of the hypotheses on which the study is based.

Coordination Through Managed Competition

One alternative is to coordinate the agencies through a managerial strategy of increasing decisional options open to the governor and his aides. This approach, which would make use of existing hierarchical arrangements, is best exemplified by the managerial orientation of the Division of the Budget.[19] Because the Division is faced with having to allocate state resources among a host of competing and often vaguely defined programs, it strives to clarify issues in order to simplify and rationalize the process of choice. There is, however, an important and crucial difference between the Division's efforts to increase rationality in decision-making and the approach to coordination being considered. The Division, and others, tend to regard the pulling and hauling among the state agencies as a pernicious reality of life that unfortunately must be lived with, a process that muddies the waters and makes matters more difficult to settle according to "objective" criteria. What is suggested here is that the competition and conflict among the agencies be recognized as a necessary and useful aspect of interorganizational life, and, further,

18. It is beyond the scope of this study to consider the many specific examples of hierarchical alternatives to the Council concept.

19. The Division's managerial approach is perhaps best reflected in recent guidelines that it has issued to state departments, presenting an integrated planning, programming, and budget system that rests heavily upon modern concepts of systems analysis. See *Guidelines for Integrated Planning-Programming-Budgeting* (Albany, N.Y., n.d.).

that it be manipulated in order to identify and clarify issues so they can be resolved more intelligently.[20]

How might this be done? The "coordinator" obviously would have to be the governor and his staff; only they possess the authority and power to manipulate the agencies. And of course the governor has legal responsibility for management of the executive branch. Although which unit of the governor's staff should oversee the process for him will not be considered here, it is visualized that the Division of the Budget would play a central role.

The coordinating process would work somewhat as follows: In the particular policy sector in which it was thought that increased coordination might be desirable, the governor (the Division of the Budget, the Governor's Secretary, etc.) would request each of the agencies affected to spell out the problem in question and suggest specific alternative proposals for meeting it. Consequently, each of the agencies would be confronted with a situation to which it would have to respond, and thus each would advance or defend its interests depending upon the probable impact of the issues. As a result each would strive assiduously to present as strong a case as possible, drawing upon available sources of information and professional knowledge.[21] The governor would then be presented with various alternative approaches to the problem, which he could evaluate and define through further requests and which he could use as a basis for acting, and hence coordinating, the agencies.

20. "Conflict may initiate other types of interaction between antagonists, even previously unrelated antagonists. It also usually takes place within a universe of norms prescribing the forms in which it is carried out. Conflict acts as a stimulus for establishing new rules, norms, and institutions, thus serving as an agent of socialization for both contending parties. Furthermore, conflict reaffirms dormant norms and intensifies participation in social life. As a stimulus for the creation and modification of norms, conflict makes the readjustment of relationships to changed conditions possible." Lewis A. Coser, *The Functions of Social Conflict* (New York, 1956), p. 128.

21. "Conflict with another group leads to the mobilization of the energies of group members and hence to increased cohesion of the group" (*ibid.*, p. 95).

Whether this approach would, however, result in satisfactory exploration of the issues involved and produce reasonable and practical alternatives for dealing with them would depend upon several factors. Much would be contingent upon the administration's ability to control the situation through the way it framed the questions placed before the agencies, and thus upon its prior knowledge of the issues. Consequently, the informational resources and technical expertise of the governor's staff would be an important factor in the success of such an approach, particularly the staff's ability to assess the agencies' performance, the state of knowledge in the field, and the relevant political considerations. Here the resources and skills of the Division of the Budget would be indispensable. But even more fundamental, as has been mentioned, the amount of coordination that could be achieved would be limited by the extent to which the policy problems at issue would be definable, for unless there is a fairly widely accepted body of knowledge about the nature of the problems and how they can be met, there are bound to be inadequate criteria for making policy choices, except on an arbitrary or political basis. If the issues could not be defined, both the governor's opportunities to control the questions put to the agencies and the agencies' ability to produce satisfactory responses would be greatly reduced.

This method of coordinating also would be useful in determining the extent to which coordination might be possible as well as desirable in a particular policy area. For example, the administration could proceed cautiously on some issues, testing to see what would be involved. It might look into the matter of whether there are accepted standards of health need and service, and what agency reactions might be if it attempted to resolve the issues. If an issue were found to be too amorphous or not politically ripe for resolution—for example, the resistance to coordination may be overwhelming—the matter could be dropped until the situation should improve.

The principal advantages of this strategy of coordinating the agencies are that it would insure the consideration of relevant points of view and values, and at the same time increase the decisional options of the governor. The strategy would seek only to impose on the agencies such policies as they have played a major part in formulating. Also, if the approach is problem-centered, opportunistic, and incremental, it would be unlikely to increase conflict among the agencies to the point that the counter-pressures generated would embarrass the governor, unless there were a miscalculation. But, in being incremental, there would be less chance of error than if coordination were attempted by a substantial centralization of authority. In addition, since only a few issues would be faced at one time, only the agencies affected and their constituents would be capable of generating counter-pressures. Furthermore, in being dealt with unilaterally and being encouraged to compete with each other, the agencies would be less able to take joint defensive measures, except for each to determine what the others might propose and then attempt to produce recommendations that would have a maximum chance of gaining acceptance.

A Reformed Council

The second modest alternative approach to coordinating the agencies would be to reestablish and reorganize the Council, for the Council could be significantly changed as an instrument of interdepartmental coordination by remedying its chief structural weakness—lack of power over its members. An obvious strategy would be to grant the Council legal authority over its members. This would be difficult and perhaps undesirable, because any authority that the Council might be given would dilute the authority of the governor and conflict with the legal responsibilities of the member agencies. To this extent, it would actually increase the difficulties of coordination within the executive branch as a whole. Consequently, the only practical alternative would be for a superordinate authority with an interest in coordinating the member agencies, such as the governor or the legislature, to manage the Council. Of these the governor would be the only appropriate choice, because of his responsibility for managing the executive branch.

For the governor to manage the Council would require that the mechanism be linked more closely to his office than it was. This could be done in several ways, which vary principally in the kind and amount of control they would provide the governor. For example, the Council could be chaired by the governor himself, or a member of his staff (Executive Chamber, Division of the Budget). The Council also could be staffed by the governor's office (Executive Chamber, Division of the Budget). In addition, the status of the staff could be raised (Executive Director instead of Executive Secretary); its role enlarged (selection of agenda items, initiation of studies, etc.); and its size and composition expanded by adding specialists in the main aspects of the functions of the member agencies.

Joining the Council to the governor's office would, however, change the Council in many ways, some profound, depending primarily upon the closeness of the union, but also on how powerful the governor might be, and how much he would attempt to manage the instrumentality. First, how the Council's basic characteristics would be affected will be discussed, without specifying any particular degree of intervention by the governor. Then consideration will be given to how management of the Council would affect its capacity to coordinate, taking into account what the governor would be likely to do and the imperatives that would influence him.

Interdepartmental politics. Depending on how high the stakes were, gubernatorial management of the Council would intensify the competition among the agencies for functions, resources, and prestige, and thus raise the political temperature of this part of the executive branch. If the Council became an important factor in the decisions made by the administration, the agencies would have considerable incentive to influence the governor in his handling of the mechanism. For example, the agencies would try to influence the issues to be brought up, the terms in which they would be presented, and the criteria by which the actions taken in the Council would be judged. In the maneuvering for position some departments would naturally fare better than others and would intensify their efforts to improve and maintain their standing with the governor. If some became strong favorites, the others would have to defer to them to some extent. Making the Council an important decision-making body also would attract the attention of the agencies' constituents and other private interest groups active in the health field in New York. Depending upon how the issues placed before the Council would affect them they, too, could be expected to watch the Council carefully and try to influence its operation through their access to the agencies, the governor, and others. Moreover, if the agencies felt it necessary, they could be expected to alert their supporters on important issues. Even the legislature would pay much more attention to the Council than it has, and it would be drawn into some issues, if it felt that the Council were impinging on its sphere of influence. This could lead to friction between the governor and the legislature.

The advantages and disadvantages of Council participation. Active involvement of the governor in the affairs of the Council would change the advantages and disadvantages experienced by the agencies in being members of the instrumentality. The agencies generally would find membership much more threatening than they now do, because the risks of participating would be greater and more difficult to calculate and control. The risks (and the potential benefits) would, however, be unevenly distributed among them, so that the agencies also would tend to value the Council differently.

The extent to which the agencies would find the benefits and costs of involvement in the Council to be different would depend upon many interrelated factors, but primarily these would be the agencies' success in influencing the governor's management of the mechanism, the governor's capacity to control the member departments, and the extent to which the vital interests of the agencies would be affected by the Council. First, a member that was consistently able to gain its ends by swaying the governor would be much less threatened than one that was not. Contingent upon how successful it was, such a member might even come to view the Council as a net advantage; however, even a very successful department would tend to be cautious in its views of the mechanism, for there would be the ever-present danger that the tables could be turned by a change in political fortunes, such as by the election of a new governor, or some unforeseen crisis. Similarly, the degree of constitutional, statutory, and political control that the governor is able to exercise over an agency would significantly affect how advantageous and disadvantageous the agency would find the Council. For example, the more autonomous the department, and the more protected it is by a powerful constituency, the less threatened it would be under a system in which the governor would be more active in Council affairs. Likewise, the more the Council would deal with matters affecting an agency's functions, the more it would consider participation disadvantageous, unless it usually had a favored position. Differences in such factors as the magnitude and relative importance of the agencies' health responsibilities, size, general outlook, and internal organizational structure therefore would play a much larger part in determining how valuable the Council would be to its members compared to the earlier Council. Consequently, the character of the Council's membership would have a greater impact upon the operation of the Council.

The informal functions of the Council. Although gubernatorial management of the Council would increase the disadvantages to the agencies participating in the mechanism, it would also increase the incentives to these agencies in cooperating to control their external environment, keeping an eye on each other to reduce the hazards of interagency competition, and discovering and exploiting areas of convergent interest among their programs. But because such management would change the character of the incentives, it would affect the Council's performance of each of these functions differently. Pressures from the governor to face up to controversial issues would make the agencies' external environment and their relations with each other more hazardous. This might increase the incentives to ameliorate the sources of trouble by exchanging information and cooperating to define and resolve the underlying issues. However, as hazards might increase, the agencies would be less likely to cooperate with each other unless it were absolutely necessary. In addition, the more that the risks of cooperating would be unevenly borne by the agencies (the extent would depend on the variables described above), the less likely they would be to cooperate, for potential winners would be more inclined to press their advantage and potential losers would be more fearful of cooperating. In such a situation the difficulty of calculating the benefits and costs of cooperating also would be greater, a fact that would reduce the predictability of behavior, a necessary condition for cooperation.

Depending upon the degree of gubernatorial pressure, therefore, and the degree to which the benefits and costs of cooperating would be unevenly distributed, the incentives to cooperate would increasingly become negative, such as accepting the governor's right to command, avoiding his displeasure, and preventing the imposition of sanctions, if the question at issue were not settled to his satisfaction. In fact, such considerations would lie at the root of the governor's ability to persuade the Council to face up to disagreements among its members. Consequently, coordination would increasingly come to depend upon "enforced" cooperation in contrast to "voluntary" cooperation.[22]

This process would affect the informal functions of the Council. As the pressures to cooperate would increase, the Council would be less capable of helping the agencies discover and exploit areas of convergent interest among their health programs, for the risks of doing so probably would be greater in performing this function than the others. Such action as the Council has taken of this kind has depended upon voluntary agreement. This does not mean that the agencies would not make changes in their programs in order to coordinate them, but that they would be less likely to do so unless they were so compelled in order to mitigate outside pressures. Next, the agencies probably would grow increasingly hesitant to exchange information and views voluntarily in order to keep watch on each other, and thus reduce the risks of injur-

22. See pp. 54–55.

ing each other needlessly outside of the Council. The risks of cooperating in this way certainly would not be as great as the dangers of working out arrangements among their programs. The agencies also would continue to learn a great deal about each other in being required by the governor to cooperate, and they probably would be much more interested in acquiring information from agency to agency than they now are because it would be more important. Finally, the member agencies probably would continue to cooperate most, although less voluntarily, in controlling their external environment, especially in mitigating threatening pressures, particularly those generated by the governor. It is likely that this would be the case because the agencies are much more dependent upon a common environment (the governor, the legislature, private interest groups, etc.) than they are upon each other. In fact, much of their dependence upon each other is a function of their dependence upon the same third parties, particularly upon the governor. Tying the Council closely to the governor's office not only would enhance this dependence, but would be the basis of such control as the governor would be able to exert over the instrumentality.

Council rules, strategies, and processes. If the Council were managed by the governor, the member agencies probably would continue to observe essentially the same informal rules. Although making the Council deal with controversial questions would increase the incentives for the agencies to push their interests regardless of expense to each other, the agencies still would probably have a surpassing interest in keeping the conflict within the Council at a minimum. First, they would seek to reach agreement by unanimous consent. Obviously, the agencies that might be outvoted would resist majority rule, because they would not want to lose or be registered as being in opposition to the others. But even the agencies in a favored position would be constrained by the realization that such a practice could be used against them in the future. Today's winners could be tomorrow's losers.[23]

23. In discussing the Council of Ministers of the European Coal and Steel Community, Ernst B. Haas reports: "The code of the council clearly demands, though the Treaty does not, that all decisions other than consul-

Permitting majority rule also would encourage the formation of coalitions, which would intensify conflict and decrease the predictability of interdepartmental relations. Moreover, an agency that benefited from Council action at another's expense would prefer to minimize the costs of its gains because of the possible need for the loser's help on other matters, or even for example in capitalizing on its immediate gains. Consequently, the more agencies would have to take each other's actions into account in acting, or the more interdependent they would be, the less likely would a majority attempt to force its will on a minority.

Similarly, the agencies probably would continue to observe the unwritten rule of not participating in decisions, unless their interests were affected, except to confirm a consensus.[24] Moreover, in instances of substantial disagreement, the parties involved probably would be expected to settle the matter themselves. Management of the Council by the governor's office would therefore lead to some bargaining over differences among the agencies, much of which probably would occur outside of the Council to protect the interests of the contending parties and to avoid embarrassing the other members. But contrary to the state of affairs under the earlier Council, the parties to the issue would be under considerable pressure to resolve the matter and bring an agree-

tations requested by the High Authority be made by unanimity. Governments knowing that binding opinions could be made in some situations despite their negative vote and that some agreement is called for in any case, are extremely unwilling to be forced into the position of being the single holdout, thus to be isolated and exposed as 'anti-European.' Governments placed in a majority position, moreover, realizing that they may at some future time be put in the place of the dissenter, prefer not to isolate their colleagues. Hence the search for unanimously acceptable decisions meeting the logic of accelerated integration goes on until a formula is found." See *The Uniting of Europe* (Stanford, 1958), p. 523.

24. In a discussion of the National Security Council, Paul Y. Hammond indicates that the Planning Board of the Council apparently "has been quite resentful of 'third party' contributions, and that in fact it has operated with unwritten rules of jurisdiction on this score which, when violated, has caused considerable friction." And he goes on to say, "There is no reason to doubt that the same pressures have operated to some degree in the Council." See "The National Security Council as a Device for Interdepartmental Coordination: An Interpretation and Appraisal," *The American Political Science Rev.*, LIV (Dec. 1960), 906.

ment back to the Council for approval as a Council decision. Left to themselves, these agencies probably would try to settle the matter at the lowest common denominator of agreement within the realities of their situation.[25] Depending upon the extent of gubernatorial interest in the issue, however, and the difficulty of resolving it, the governor's office might participate in the negotiations. Generally the parties involved would prefer to avoid having others help settle their differences, which would give them added incentive to work out an understanding. But, depending upon how much their interests were at stake, the agencies would welcome the support of their constituents and other interest groups—their involvement probably could not be avoided, if the latter felt their interests were at issue—to bring pressure upon the governor, the Council, and others. In this way the conflict might spread and thereby embarrass the governor and one or more of the agencies.

Although compelling the Council to deal with controversial questions would lead to bargaining among its members, the agencies, insofar as they could, probably would try to handle matters on which they disagreed by analytic processes (persuasion and problem-solving) instead of bargaining.[26] They would do so in order to avoid the cost of bargaining, such as acknowledgement of victory and defeat—a better bargain for one would be a poor one for another—and the accompanying embarrassment. Thus, for example, there would be increased incentive to define and settle disagreements in noncontroversial terms. And for the same reasons, the agencies would engage in processes of mutual

25. Paul Hammond also reports that the Planning Board of the National Security Council has been criticized on the grounds that it "in its pursuit of 'common grounds,' is inclined to 'plaster over' significant issues and differences with carefully chosen ambiguities, or language plagued with equivocations expressive of the lowest common denominator of agreement. In the NSC itself as well, it is claimed, there is a reluctance to exacerbate differences of view and opinion, with the result that discussion is inclined to be more courteous than probing" (*ibid.*, p. 904).

26. See pp. 128–31.

adjustment not involving face-to-face encounters.[27] For example, they would be more inclined to bargain tacitly, in which the "adversaries watch and interpret each other's behavior, each aware that his actions are being interpreted and anticipated, each acting with a view to the expectations that he creates";[28] however, when these modes of behavior proved inadequate—for example, if the parties were too far apart—explicit bargaining would occur.

To gain their ends the agencies also would make greater use of offensive and defensive strategies than they did in the past. In contrast to the former relaxed atmosphere of Council meetings, in which aggressive agencies easily could be checked, Council deliberations would become more highly charged. Since the opportunities to gain a relative advantage would be greater, there would be more in-fighting within the Council's informal rules.[29] Although this would put much greater strain on the rules, it is unlikely that the agencies in an advantageous position would violate them much more than they formerly did, for they would still lose more than they would gain by not observing them. The strategies employed by the agencies would however be more highly developed, particularly the ways of influencing the Council through the governor and other third parties.

What a restructured Council could do. How much coordination the Council could accomplish would depend mainly upon the extent to which governors would be managing it and how they would do so, which would, of course, depend upon the consequences that the mechanism would have for the gubernatorial

27. Though many of the types of mutual adjustment that he defines customarily have been treated as bargaining (explicit and tacit), Charles Lindblom also identifies other types of "adaptive" and "manipulated" adjustments. See Lindblom, pp. 35–84.

28. Thomas C. Schelling, *The Strategy of Conflict* (Cambridge, Mass., 1963), p. 21. See also pp. 129–31, this volume.

29. "Interdependence [of groups], while checking tendencies toward a radical break with the system, is no bar to differences of interest leading to conflict; on the contrary, the greater the interdependence, the sharper the focus upon questions of relative advantage." Coser, p. 76.

office. Tying the Council closely to the governor's office not only would increase its capacity to coordinate its members, but also would bring about changes in Council operation and in the character of interdepartmental relations that would have costs as well as benefits.

Because of the disadvantages, it is unlikely that the governor would push the Council very far, particularly because of the intensification of competition among the member agencies that would result, thereby increasing the pressures on the chief executive and the risks that controversies might get out of hand. No governor would knowingly attempt to resolve a controversy, if there were a good chance of the costs becoming excessive, as this would weaken his authority and probably his political position as well. Moreover, any governor would be concerned about the possibility that the agencies and their constituents might try to use the Council to present a united front against him on some matters, and thus reduce his options, which of course it would have greater incentive to do. Even though the Council still could only advise him, the governor could not stand in the way of its offering unsolicited advice he might nevertheless have to accept, at least in part.

Yet, notwithstanding these dangers, the Council would have a number of advantages that might encourage the governor to make some use of it. Even though his active involvement in the Council would lead to efforts to influence his management of the instrumentality, the Council would increase his opportunities to resolve controversial interdepartmental questions in professional and technical terms, or under conditions of controlled bargaining, provided of course that he did not push the instrumentality too hard. In other words, the Council could be helpful in defining some issues in nonpolitical terms, which would make them somewhat easier to resolve and would afford the governor greater control over their resolution. The Council also would be helpful to the governor in deflecting some public pressures from himself. For example, if an issue were one that could reasonably be interpreted in professional terms, as many health issues are, he could refer it to the Council and thereby put the pressure on his department heads to come up with a solution. Moreover, the Council would be useful to the governor as a sounding board in testing departmental reactions to possible moves on his part. The Council might even prevent the development of some controversies by helping the governor and the agencies in identifying them in their nascent stages when they are easier to resolve.

How much coordinating the Council could do also would depend upon how closely the governor participated in its management. If he turned to the Council on matters it could well handle, and kept abreast of its activities, it would become an important locus of decision-making capable of dealing with fundamental issues of state policy. Although the governor obviously would want to permit his department heads direct access to his office, a great deal would depend on how much he accomplished through other channels. Likewise, although he would respect and trust some of his commissioners more than others, much also would depend upon how responsive he was to their attempts to circumvent the Council by means of their access to him. Consequently, the governor's personal outlook and style of operation, including the way in which he related to his confidants and subordinates, would strongly color the Council.

However, the more closely it was identified with the governor, the more uncertain the Council's future would be. Since governors inevitably vary in their outlook and other attributes, the instrumentality probably would change radically with each new administration, and might not survive at all. Indeed the member agencies, at least those that fared most poorly, probably would encourage a new governor to bring about the Council's demise. Attaching the Council too closely to the governor's immediate office also would make it more difficult to develop an expert staff that could hold its own with the commissioners and their top aides, as the staff probably would change with each change in administration.

Furthermore, there is no way of institutionalizing the Council without making sacrifices in its ability to deal with sensitive matters, because this requires creating some distance between the governor and the mechanism and causes a reduction in Council power. Moreover, the element of state government to which the Council would be anchored and would derive its security also would influence Council action, as its own maintenance and enhancement needs would be brought into play. There is no way of assuring the Council's survival, except as it is valuable to the interested parties, particularly the governor. For example, if the Council were staffed outside of the governor's immediate office (Executive Chamber)—say by the Division of the Budget—it would be less able to deal with controversial matters, for the Division lacks the power of the executive chamber and would have to consider the implications of its role for the performance of regular functions. As a result, the Division would try to steer the Council in the direction of its interests in efficient allocation and management of state resources. Depending therefore upon how much the Division was able to influence it, the Council would tend to be concerned with reconciling agency program plans and improving the administrative relationships among the agencies' programs, matters about which the Council has done little. By contrast, the governor would tend to be more interested in developing new programs with public appeal and resolving interagency conflicts that were a burden to his administration.

Probably the most satisfactory way of restructuring the Council would be for a top aide of the governor, such as a special assistant for Council affairs, to chair the Council, and have the Division of the Budget provide the staffing. This arrangement would give the Council the strength of the governor's immediate office and the stability and expertise of the Division of the Budget. It also would tend to optimize the Council's capacity to deal with both the policy and administrative aspects of the relationships among the member agencies. Certainly such a council would be better able to increase coordination of the agencies than the former mechanism. Moreover, because of the constraints that would be inherent in its operation, it seems likely that the benefits would exceed the costs for the governor and his constituents, the people of New York.

In Conclusion

It seems clear that greater interdepartmental coordination cannot be achieved by a mechanism such as the Interdepartmental Health and Hospital Council. Moreover, only two basic alternatives are possible to a coordinating council that cannot be granted authority: namely, coordination by hierarchy and coordination by a council managed by an authority superior to the member agencies, which presupposes the existence of such an authority.[30] Certainly the latter method deserves serious consideration in organizational design, as the foregoing discussion indicates. In many situations the most satisfactory solution may lie in optimizing the advantages of coordination by hierarchy and coordination by council.[31] Such an arrangement may convert the major weakness of councils into a strength—their having to come to terms with the maintenance and enhancement needs of their members—for a reasonable regard for such needs is important to accomplishment, especially when top professional performance is required. Moreover, a reformed council certainly would give the agencies a greater voice in the process of coordination than the alternative of increasing the policy options of the governor through stimulating interagency competition. Consequently, it also would place greater reliance upon decision-making through compromise and mutual adjustments among the agencies than on choosing from among clearly defined policy alternatives. But which of these or other alternatives would be preferable in any given situation cannot be determined unless the need for coordination is defined and until more studies are made of different organizational arrangements.

30. One obvious hierarchical solution would be to create a superdepartment, such as a department of health, education, and welfare. This would, however, require basic constitutional changes in New York and would create new problems of coordination, although of an intradepartmental character.

31. In his review of the National Security Council, Paul Hammond concludes: "In the end, the question of how best to achieve interdepartmental coordination of national security policy must be answered by weighing these two major alternatives against each other [NSC type of council or a presidential staff], or by finding the optimum mixture of them." See Hammond, p. 910.

APPENDIX, BIBLIOGRAPHY, INDEX

Appendix

Procedures for Classifying Rehabilitation Issues

ALL of the rehabilitation issues that came up in the Council (Council proper and the Committee on Rehabilitation) during the period from May 1953, the date of the first meeting of the Committee on Rehabilitation, through December 1964, were classified according to the characteristics described below. The information needed to determine these characteristics was obtained through the methods of the study described in Chapter 1, pages 21–23, in particular through review of the records of the Council (agenda, minutes, reports, etc.) and interviews of state officials and other persons familiar with the issues and the Council's handling of them. Many decisions regarding the classification of specific issues also were checked with the staff of the Council and with others as well. Nevertheless, considerable judgment has been exercised in classifying the issues because of the impreciseness of the criteria employed.

Definition of an Issue

An issue is a question affecting one or more of the Council agencies requiring some kind of decision for its resolution. When brought before the Council, an issue became an agenda item. However, since an issue may last for several years, it may have involved many agenda items. In considering an issue in the Council, the member agencies could either take some kind of joint action to resolve it (a decision) or not (no decision).

Characteristics of Issues

The rehabilitation issues that came up at Council meetings (the Council proper or the Committee on Rehabilitation) were classified according to the following attributes:

Subject. The subject of each issue is its unique substantive character. Since some of the issues were interrelated and blended into each other it was sometimes difficult to distinguish them without some arbitrariness. However, insofar as possible, the substantive nature of the issue as seen by the participating agencies has been used as the criterion. This approach has the advantage of keeping the analysis as close to reality as possible. Altogether, 64 different issues have been identified.

Initiator. The initiator is the agency or group that refers the issue to the Council (to the chairman or staff of the Council proper or the Committee on Rehabilitation). An initiator may, of course, be prompted by a third party. No attempt has been made, however, to study the motivation of the referring agency or group, except where it clearly was acting as an agent. The object was to identify the agency that for whatever purpose tried to initiate the decision-making process by presenting the issue to the Council.

Life of an issue. The life of an issue in the Council is the length of time between the date it was first received and the last date it was considered there. Generally, the beginning date is the first time the issue was presented to a meeting of the Council (Council proper or the Committee on Rehabilitation), except if it was communicated in writing to the Council. The ending date is less precise. Except for decisions implying some kind of follow-up by the Council, it is the date the issue was last considered. In the case of an issue in which there was some follow-up, the terminal date is the date of the last meeting at which progress was reported. Hence considerable arbitrariness has entered into determining the life of issues. Also, an issue need not have been considered continuously, but may have lain dormant for many meetings, only to be revived again at a later date.

Functional implications of an issue. The functional implications of an issue are: (1) whether it was brought up in the Council as a result of environmental pressure, particularly whether it was referred to the Council by an outside group (the governor, private interest group, etc.) or brought up voluntarily by a member agency as a result of specific pressures felt outside of the Council, and therefore, whether the issue involved mitigating external pressure; (2) whether the issue was initiated by a member agency in the absence of environmental pressures, and thus, whether it primarily involved taking the initiative to influence groups in the agencies' external environment or to work out arrangements among their programs. This schema made it possible to obtain some quantitative measure of the relative importance of the informal functions that the Council performed for its members.

Agencies interested in the issue. The agencies interested in an issue are those whose interests were most affected by its consideration in the Council, and hence also are the agencies that were most active in the disposition of the issue.

Controversiality. An issue was labeled controversial, and thus involved conflict, if one or more of the members felt strongly that it could not be resolved without another member gaining at its (the first agency's) expense, or if in being acted upon by the Council this result would occur.

Transfer of Functions. An issue potentially involved a transfer of functions, or responsibilities from one agency to another, if one or more agencies thought that its resolution might require such action, and actually did if a Council decision called for such action. Whether the transfer of functions actually occurred as a consequence of Council action is still another question.

Legislative change. An issue potentially involved legislative action if the agencies felt that its resolution might require such action, and actually did if a Council decision called for such action. Again, whether legislation was enacted as a result of Council action is another question.

Exchange of resources. An issue potentially involved an exchange of resources among the member agencies (funds, manpower, clients, etc.), if such a result was implicit or explicit in the action taken by the Council, and actually did if the action of the Council contributed to this result, at least in part.

Bibliography

Books

Banfield, Edward C. *Political Influence.* New York: The Free Press, 1961.

Blau, Peter M. and W. Richard Scott. *Formal Organizations.* San Francisco: Chandler Publishing Co., 1962.

Braybrooke, David and Charles E. Lindblom. *A Strategy of Decision.* New York: The Free Press, 1963.

Caldwell, Lynton K. *The Government and Administration of New York.* American Commonwealth Series. New York: Thomas Y. Crowell, 1954.

Coser, Lewis A. *The Functions of Social Conflict.* New York: The Free Press, 1956.

Fox, Irving and Isabel Picken. *The Upstream-Downstream Controversy in the Arkansas-White-Red Basin Survey.* The Inter-University Case Series, No. 55. University, Ala.: University of Alabama Press, 1960.

Friedrich, Carl J. *Constitutional Government and Politics.* New York and London: Harper, 1937.

Gross, Bertram M. *The Managing of Organizations.* 2 vols. New York: The Free Press, 1964.

Haas, Ernest B. *The Uniting of Europe.* Stanford: Stanford University Press, 1958.

Herzberg, Donald G. and Paul Tillett. *A Budget for New York State, 1956–57.* The Inter-University Case Series, No. 69. University, Alabama: University of Alabama Press, 1962.

Homans, George C. *The Human Group.* New York: Harcourt, Brace & Co., 1950.

Hyman, Herbert H., Charles R. Wright, and Terrence K. Hopkins. *Applications of Methods of Evaluation.* Berkeley and Los Angeles: University of California Press, 1962.

Lindblom, Charles E. *The Intelligence of Democracy.* New York: The Free Press, 1965.

March, James G. and Herbert A. Simon. *Organizations.* New York: John Wiley and Sons, 1958.

Merton, Robert K. *Social Theory and Social Structure.* Revised ed. New York: The Free Press, 1957.

Mott, Basil J. F. *Financing and Operating Rehabilitation Centers and Facilities.* Chicago: National Society for Crippled Children and Adults, 1960.

Novick, David (ed.). *Program Budgeting.* Cambridge: Harvard University Press, 1965.

Polyani, Michael. *The Logic of Liberty.* Chicago: University of Chicago Press, 1951.

Prethus, Robert. *The Organizational Society.* New York: Vintage Books, 1965.

Sayles, Leonard R. *Managerial Behavior.* New York: McGraw-Hill Book Co., 1964.

Sayre, Wallace S. and Herbert Kaufman. *Governing New York City.* New York: Russell Sage Foundation, 1960.

Schelling, Thomas C. *The Strategy of Conflict.* Cambridge: Harvard University Press, 1963.

Selznick, Philip. *TVA and the Grass Roots.* Berkeley and Los Angeles: University of California Press, 1953.

Sills, David L. *The Volunteers.* New York: The Free Press, 1957.

Straetz, Ralph A. and Frank J. Munger. *New York Politics.* Prepared under the auspices of The Citizenship Clearing House. New York: New York University Press, 1960.

Thompson, Victor A. *Modern Organization.* New York: Alfred A. Knopf, 1961.

Trackett, Mary Fitzmaurice (Reynolds). *Interdepartmental Committees in the National Administration.* New York: Columbia University Press, 1939.

Tullock, Gordon. *The Politics of Bureaucracy.* Washington, D. C.: Public Affairs Press, 1965.

Vidich, Arthur J. and Joseph Bensman. *Small Town in Mass Society.* Garden City: Doubleday (Anchor Books), 1960.

Wildavsky, Aaron B. *The Politics of the Budgetary Process.* Boston: Little, Brown and Co., 1964.

Articles in Collections

Dimock, Marshall E. "Expanding Jurisdictions: A Case Study in Bureacratic Conflict," in *Reader in Bureaucracy,* ed. Robert K. Merton, et al. New York: The Free Press, 1952.

Gouldner, Alvin W. "Organizational Analysis," in *Sociology Today,* ed. Robert K. Merton, Leonard Broom, and Leonard S. Cottrell, Jr. New York: Basic Books, 1959.

Haire, Mason. "Biological Models and Empirical Histories of the Growth of Organizations," in *Modern Organization Theory*, ed. Mason Haire. New York: John Wiley and Sons, 1959.

Thompson, James D. and William J. McEwen. "Organizational Goals and Environment," in *Complex Organizations, A Sociological Reader*, ed. Amitai Etzioni. New York: Holt, Rinehart, and Winston, 1961.

Wilson, James Q. in "Innovation in Organization: Notes Toward a Theory," in *Approaches to Organizational Design*, ed. James D. Thompson. Pittsburgh, Pa.: University of Pittsburgh Press, 1966.

Articles

Bell, James R. "A Coordinator for State Government Agencies," *Public Administration Review*, XVIII (Spring 1958), 98–101.

Bradley, Phillips. "Interlocking Collaboration in Albany," *Public Administration Review*, XVII (Summer 1957), 180–87.

Brightman, I. Jay. "An Interdepartmental Approach to Health," *Public Health Reports*, LXXIII (October 1958), 919–24.

————. "Problems in Interdisciplinary Coordination and Communication," *Annals of The New York Academy of Sciences*, LXXIV (September 1958), 35–39.

Clark, Peter B. and James Q. Wilson. "Incentives Systems: A Theory of Organizations," *Administrative Science Quarterly*, VI (September 1961), 129–66.

Etzioni, Amitai. "New Directions in the Study of Organizations and Society," *Social Research*, XXVII (Summer 1960), 223–28.

Fenton, Joseph. "Interdepartmental Coordination of Rehabilitation in New York State Government," *Rehabilitation Literature*, XXV (April 1964), 98–104, 112.

Friedman, Robert S., Bernard S. Klein, and John H. Romani, "Administrative Agencies and the Publics They Serve," *Public Administration Review*, XXVI (September 1966), 192–204.

Gouldner, Alvin W. "Cosmopolitans and Locals: Toward an Analysis of Latent Social Roles, I, II," *Administrative Science Quarterly*, II (December 1957 and March 1958), 281–306 and 444–80.

Guetzkow, Harold. "Interagency Committee Usage," *Public Administration Review*, X (Summer 1960), 190–96.

Hammond, Paul Y. "The National Security Council as a Device for Interdepartmental Coordination: An Interpretation and Appraisal," *The American Political Science Review*, LIV (December 1960), 899–910.

Kaufman, Herbert. "Emerging Conflicts in the Doctrines of Public Administration," *The American Political Science Review*, L (December 1956), 1057–73.

Levine, Sol and Paul E. White. "Exchange as a Conceptual Framework for the Study of Interorganizational Relationships," *Administrative Science Quarterly*, V (March 1961), 583–601.

Litwak, Eugene and Lydia F. Hylton. "Interorganizational Analysis: A Hypothesis on Coordinating Agencies," *Administrative Science Quarterly*, VI (March 1962), 398–420.

Miller, Walter B. "Inter-Institutional Conflict as a Major Impedient to Delinquency Prevention," *Human Organization*, XVII (Fall 1958), 20–23.

Musicus, Milton. "Reappraising Reorganization," *Public Administrative Review*, XXIV (June 1964), 107–12.

Schlesinger, Edward R. "A New Program for the Rehabilitation of the Handicapped," *American Journal of Public Health*, LIII, No. 3 (March 1963), 398–402.

Thompson, James D. "Organizations and Output Transactions," *The American Journal of Sociology*, LXVIII (November 1962), 309–24.

Zander, Alvin and Donald Wolfe. "Administrative Rewards and Coordination Among Committee Members," *Administrative Science Quarterly*, IX (June 1964), 50–70.

New York State Documents

COUNCIL PAPERS

Minutes of the Interdepartmental Health Council (IHC), 1953–1956.

Minutes of the Interdepartmental Health Resources Board (IHRB), 1956–1960.

Minutes of the Interdepartmental Health and Hospital Council (IHHC), 1960–1966.

Minutes of the Committee on Rehabilitation of the IHC, 1953–1956, the IHRB, 1956–1960, and the IHHC, 1960–1966.

Minutes of Joint Meeting of the Governor's Council on Rehabilitation and the IHHC, May 29, 1961.

Recommendations from Sub-Committee on Coordination of School and Community Health Services, July, 1948. Exhibit 4, attached to the Agenda, IHC meeting, February 1, 1950.

Proposal for the Improvement of Nursing Education and Service. Albany: Interdepartment Health Council of New York State, December 1950.

Memorandum from Dr. Herman E. Hilleboe [Chairman, IHC] to Hon. Averell Harriman. Interdepartmental Council on Human Resources, February 21, 1955.

New York State Program in Rehabilitation. A Report by the Board Committee on Rehabilitation to the Interdepartmental Health Resources Board. Albany: Interdepartmental Health Resources Board, December 1, 1959.

Report of the Sub-Committee to Determine the IHHC Rehabilitation Committee Responsibility for Probationers, Parolees, and Prisoners, February 6, 1964. See Exhibit III, Minutes of the Committee on Rehabilitation, January 20, 1964.

GOVERNOR'S PAPERS

"Message Submitting a Comprehensive Public Health Program, March 4, 1946," *Public Papers of Governor Thomas E. Dewey, 1946.* Albany, n.d.

"Statement–Appointment of Interdepartmental Health Council, October 5, 1946," *Public Papers of Governor Thomas E. Dewey, 1946.* Albany, n.d.

"Appointments, Interdepartmental Health Council, September 22, 1953," *Public Papers of Governor Thomas E. Dewey, 1953.* Albany, n.d.

"Message Concerning Public Health and Mental Health, January 17, 1956," *Public Papers of Governor W. Averell Harriman, 1956.* Albany, n.d.

Message of Governor Nelson A. Rockefeller to the Legislature, January 7, 1959. Legislative Document No. 1. Albany, 1959.

Proposed Reorganization of the Executive Branch of New York State Government, Report to Governor Nelson A. Rockefeller. Albany, December 1959.

"Message Recommending a Rehabilitation Program for Disabled Citizens of the State, March 16, 1959," *Public Papers of Governor Nelson A. Rockefeller, 1959.* Albany, n.d.

"Executive Order Establishing an Interdepartmental Health and Hospital Council, March 31, 1960," *Public Papers of Governor Nelson A. Rockefeller, 1960.* Albany, n.d.

New York State Organization Study of State Rehabilitation Services, Office of Secretary to the Governor, October 1960.

Press Release of Governor Nelson A. Rockefeller, October 17, 1960. Albany.

Message of Governor Nelson A. Rockefeller to the Legislature, January 3, 1962. Legislative Document No. 1. Albany, 1962.

"Message Presenting a Comprehensive New Master Plan in Aid of the Mentally Disabled, January 30, 1962," *Public Papers of Governor Nelson A. Rockefeller, 1962*. Albany, n.d.

Letter from Governor Nelson A. Rockefeller to Dr. Herman E. Hilleboe and the Honorable Thomas Thacher, Interdepartmental Health and Hospital Council. Albany, October 12, 1962.

OTHER PAPERS

Temporary Legislative Commission to Formulate a Long Range State Health Program, *Medical Care in New York State, 1939*, Legislative Document No. 91. Albany, 1940.

New York State Legislative Commission on Medical Care, *Medical Care for the People of New York*. Albany, February 15, 1946.

Memorandum from Dr. Hilleboe to Members of Interdepartmental Councils and Commissions, Reorganization of Councils, Commissions, and Committees, November 7, 1952.

Memorandum from Clark Ahlberg, Deputy Director, to Jonathan Bingham, Secretary to the Governor, September 11, 1957.

Report to the Governor from Governor's Council on Rehabilitation. Enclosed with letter from Leonard W. Mayo, Chairman, to the Honorable Nelson A. Rockefeller, December 21, 1959.

Prepayment for Medical and Dental Care in New York State, Submitted by School of Public Health and Administrative Medicine, Columbia University, to Hon. Herman E. Hilleboe, Commissioner of Health, and Hon. Thomas Thacher, Superintendent of Insurance, October, 1962.

Public Welfare in the State of New York. Albany: Moreland Commission, January 15, 1963.

A Plan for a Comprehensive Mental Health and Mental Retardation Program for New York State. Vol. 1, Report of the Mental Health and Mental Retardation Sections of the State Planning Committee. Albany: Department of Mental Hygiene, July 1965.

U.S. Government Documents

U. S. Congress, Senate. *Organizing for National Security*. Inquiry of the Subcommittee on the National Policy Machinery, Committee on Government Operations, 86th and 87th Congresses, 1960–61. Vol. 1, Hearings, Vol. 2, Studies and Background Material, Vol. 3, Staff Reports and Recommendations.

Unpublished Material

Bobilin, Adah Dorothy. "The New York Interdepartmental Health Council." Unpublished Master's thesis, Syracuse University, 1957.

Clark, Peter B. "The Business Corporation as a Political Order." Paper presented at the 1961 Annual Meeting of the American Political Science Association, St. Louis, Missouri, September 7–9, 1961. (Mimeographed.)

Lerner, Ray. "Interdepartmental Coordination in the City of New York, A Case Study, The Interdepartmental Health Council," December, 1962. (Typewritten.)

Schaefer, Morris. "Area and Function in the Administration of Public Health in New York State." Unpublished doctoral dissertation, Syracuse University, 1962.

Index